AF881350

Adolfo Panfili

ORTHOMOLECULAR BIOHACKING BIBLE

FROM PAULING TO PANFILI

Copyright © 2025 by
Adolfo Panfili

ALL RIGHTS RESERVED. NO part of this book may be reproduced or transmitted in any form by any means, electronic or mechanical, including photocopying and recording, or by any information storage and retrieval system, except as may be expressly permitted in writing from the author.

Paperback: 978-1-964898-71-1

Hardcover: 978-1-964898-76-6

Published by:
Pine Book Writing
www.PineBookWriting.com
R-10225 Yonge St Suite #250, Richmond Hill, ON L4C 3B2, Canada.

Printed in the United States of America

LINUS PAULING INSTITUTE of SCIENCE and MEDICINE
440 Page Mill Road, Palo Alto, California 94306-2025
Telephone: (415) 327-4064
Facsimile: (415) 327-8564

28 June 1993

Dear Dr Panfili and Associates:

I am surely pleased that you have taken the initiative to form an International Association of Orthomolecular Physicians. I think that this organization can contribute a great deal to improving the health of people all over the world.

With the repeated expression to you of my thanks, and with best wishes, I am

Sincerely yours,

Linus Pauling

LP:dm

This book contains QR CODES linked to videos pertaining to the topics covered. To scan a QR CODE, the user must open the camera on their Apple iPhone or the scanner on their Android de-vice and point it at the code to access its contents.

Presentation of the work by the author

The Archangel Michael

Michael means "who resembles God" or "who is like God,"
which implies a likeness, most likely of character.
The word "archangel" is a transliteration
of the Greek archangelos.
The term combines "archon," which means "chief,"
and "angelos," which translates to "messenger" or "angel."

SUMMARY

To all those people
who have flooded
my life with enthusiasm

Why you must read this book?

The book you have chosen and are browsing through is not the effect of coincidence but of a correspondence as Charles Baudelaire stated in *Les fleurs du mal...*

Why do you read this valuable handbook?

Essentially to improve and increase the perception and awareness of one's quality of life.

This text not only removes many «VEILS» but also fulfills with rigor and dedication the goal of promoting ethical and scientific research and all-around interdisciplinary synergies.

A text for tackling the transcendant journey of rediscovering one's true self by HACKING (it really should be said) the sacred fire of the gods.

In the history of Western culture, Prometheus can be seen as a symbol of rebellion and defiance, of authority or imposition, as well as a metaphor for thought and an archetype of knowledge freed from the constraints of myth, falsification, and ideology. Novelli Prometheus the biohackers challenge obsolete and crystallized thinking with courage and enthusiasm.

This text is nimble and sober and is a pleasant read; masterfully written as Prof. Panfili does so well, and it engages the reader into the emotional and speculative dynamics that have taken place between him and multiple Nobel laureate Prof. Linus Pauling.

Prof. Panfili, as a brilliant and empathetic disciple, has developed, in more than 40 years of international medical profession the basis of future interdisciplinary synergies from which the metaphor of **Orthomolecular Biohacking** springs today. The passing of an ideal baton connecting these two men in the shared dynamic projection of improving the quality of life of humankind, not only medically, but also psychologically - spiritual.

Numerous celebrities such as heads of state, politicians, athletes, actors, (Djokovic, Morgan Freeman, Sugar, De Laurentis, Berlusconi, Keanu Reeves, etc.) have turned to this charismatic doctor/scientist to solve situations related to quality of life.

A pioneer in robotic surgery, the proper use of ADSCs (adipose tissue-derived stem cells), an experienced and seasoned clinician with a flair for teaching and communication and training, he founded the world's first faculty of NATUROPATHY AND ECO FRIENDLY ORTHOMOLECOLAR SCIENCES, commissioned by Prof. Giuseppe Sabato, a pioneer of Naturopathy at the University of Arezzo. The author of this veritable medical manual to Biohacking has more than 25 texts to his credit published in several languages (from Spanish, to English, to Korean, etc.) that represent the corpus of the Orthomolecular Biohacking approach today.
Dear Heroes: I wish you a PLEASANT JOURNEY with the wish to hack using the orthomolecular modality, changing your life for the better.

L. O.

Preface

Sir dr. prof. **Gabriele Andreoli**

scholar of complex adaptive systems, strategic consultant, analyst, writer, interdisciplinary researcher, president of the "Institute for Advance Studies and Cooperation" is a member of the American Society of Diplomacy and Political Science; Researcher and Honorary Professor at the Catholic University of New Spain, Miami, USA, Academic of Social Sciences at IASS, Florida, USA. In 2022, for his scientific commitment and faith, he was appointed Knight of the Order of St. Gregory the Great in the Vatican by the Holy Father. He received the "Future Innovation Summit Award" (Dubai) for two consecutive editions in 2022 for "cybersecurity" and in 2023 as founder of "Evolutionary Biohacking", a philosophy and research protocol for cell regeneration. In 2023, he received the "Dobrici" medal from the mayor of the city of Wieliczka for his commitment to Ukrainian refugees. For his contribution to scientific progress, he re-ceived the "Miner's Axe" (Barda górncza) award from Poland the same year. Andreoli in 2023 was named by the magazine "The Monaco Voice" as one of the most influential figures in the field of scientific research and dissemination, awarding him the "Monaco 40 over 40" awardhttps://monacovoice.com/en/article/gabriele-andreoli; founder and director of the World Changers Summit, held every year at the Pontifical Academy of Sciences in the Vatican, brings together the best minds in the field of scientific research. For his work and dedication he has received many awards including: Knight with plaque of the Sacred Military Constantinian Order of St. George, silver medal of the Italian Red Cross, silver medal of the Red Cross of San Marino, EU medal mission EUMM/Georgia, United Nations Service Medal mission UNMIK Kosovo, Commander of the Grand Cross of the Royal Order of Danilo I, Commander of the Grand Cross of Saints Maurice and Lazarus, Commander with plaque of St. Michael of the wing (Portugal)

I welcome those who are ready to read this excellent book, which will allow us to better our way of life, perception, and understanding; a statement that I have carefully considered and responsibly analyzed. As president of the "Institute for Advance Studies and Cooperation," I am responsible for promoting and carrying out ethical and scientific research, as well as creating multidisciplinary synergistic moments of contemplation. This is why, with the foundation I chair, the Institute for Advance Studies and Cooperation, we established the "World Changers Summit," which takes place annually at the Pontifical Academy of Sciences. As the originator of "Evolutionary Biohacking" in 2018, I am extremely critical of everything linked to the current management of medicine and its allied fields, such as wellness, performance medicine, ophthalmology, and so on. For me, who has studied and dealt with cell regeneration, well-being, and "performance medicine" for almost forty years, prevention remains the cornerstone of well-being and human evolution, despite the fact that little or no action is taken. I have thus consented, and I am honored, to write this brief introduction only after having had the chance to study and make my own the material contained in the book you are about to read, and I am confident that the effects of this reading will be a period of crucial contemplation. Throughout my life, I've had the privilege of working with many wonderful individuals on projects that took many scientific courses but were always connected by a common goal: to enhance people's quality of life. Today, it is more important than ever to renounce some utilitarian procedures that poison minds, bodies, and the environment. Despite significant advances in science and technology's understanding of the man/planet system, diseases (physical and psychological) have emerged in recent years, owing primarily to an incorrect interpretation of the human dimension and its relationship with technologies, medicine, and the environment.

This involution process has been facilitated, particularly in recent years, by a decline in moral and ethical values in favor of financial speculation, which has obscured the founding virtues of civil society, paving the way for poor nutrition and unhealthy habits that have weakened modern man's mind and body.

The inadequacies of many politicians, along with governments' complete lack of readiness to manage a global catastrophe, did the rest. The most recent big events that have affected a huge portion of the earth have caused us to think on the urgent need to explore new avenues for human well-being and progress, as well as the protection of our environment. Nothing happens by chance: the more you get into the research, the more you comprehend systems and our evolution, the more evident this term becomes. Let's repeat: nothing happens by chance. If you are holding this book in your hands and embarking on this trip, you will realize that this is the only time it has to happen.

Our becoming is a systemic emergent phenomena, and as such, it is the product of the whole's manifestation of creation. Concepts are wide, deep, and sophisticated tools that, when used correctly by talented minds, allow us to progress. I hope that these words will pique the reader's interest, not surprise him, but rather provide him with fresh ideas and fuel for contemplation.

I also think that everything—frustration, surprise, discouragement, enthusiasm, and misunderstandings—can be turned to our benefit if we know how to persevere. Different forces are always required and prodromal, and even if opposing, if fully utilized, they can contribute to the end result. Different forces are always required and prodromal, and even when opposing, if fully utilized, they can contribute to the end result. In saying this, I like to think of the evolution of sailing boats: once upon a time, the headwind was an insurmountable obstacle for Roman cargo ships, but with the development of dinghies and the improvement of sail, it was possible to tighten the wind even more and go, as they say in jargon, upwind, that is, upwind with edges and increasingly narrow angles. This simple example should make us think about how a result is frequently the sum of synergistic multidisciplinary talents. We must consequently keep a fiery, competent, elastic, and cooperative mentality.

I worked with biohacking before it was given this name, and I still believe that only now, thanks to the intervention of artificial intelligence, the internet, technological platforms, and new technologies of physical and chemical analysis of organic matter and its interactions with frequencies and photons, can we truly talk about biohacking.

Protocols are critical: we must control the chemicals and methods at our disposal to ensure that they are digested and used correctly by the various organs and systems in accordance with our demands and desires. I believe that biohacking requires the ability to do genetic and genomic analyses and understand their true influence and impact on the system. The potential of instantaneous feedback on the whole system of the human organism creates a difference in comparison to the past, with technologies that allow us to have clinical data on the patient under examination in real time. Of course, another intriguing aspect and cause for comparison is the interpretation and application of data. In conclusion, while we are still far from having a simple solution for everything, I feel obligated to advise individuals in the sector to rely on scientific evidence and extensive expertise. Let us avoid becoming and relying on "keyboard specialists."

Let us not be enthralled by empirical and simplistic remedies, miraculous drugs, or, most importantly, the promises of last-minute gurus who, having found biohacking in the past three or four years, claim to apply it with technology instruments whose operation and consequences they do not truly comprehend. Door-to-door snake oil salesmen who, fueled by the sensationalism of new technologies that are frequently ineffectual (especially because they are used incorrectly), generate false myths and do significant damage for the express aim of profiting and gaining celebrity.

We are aware that incorrect or inadequate diets, sedentary lifestyles, fear, stress, exposure to pollutants, radiation, and so on all contribute to the weakening of the mind and body, as well as the loss of a social goal, leaving many people without the propelling and proactive energy that is the foundation of life. Furthermore, the rapid development of goods, supplements, and "do-it-yourself" technology causes confusion and results in uncertainty. For example, while I feel that Omega 3 is beneficial in general, if we do not do specific clinical research, we will not know how and when it is metabolized, or whether there is an actual lack and why. It becomes evident that supplements can vary greatly in their efficacy for the same chemical. It is not enough to understand their quality; rather, the manner in which you consume supplements is critical, depending on how the various components are mixed. An important component of all of this is the individual's mental state: it influences the control of numerous bodily processes, but the contrary is also true. Many substances and processes also have a significant impact on the mental state. I like to believe that our intellect can perceive the human being as a cosmos of constellations and interactions, an organism composed of 10% genetics and 90% aliens: fungus, viruses, and bacteria.

The mitochondria, the cell's energetic heart, originated as a virus. The miracle of evolution is in its capacity to include what is useful. The "microbiome project," which studies interactions, is helping us understand how we might live better. Understanding our biology and how it works teaches us moral lessons about cohabitation and respect.

We must learn to behave like a foresighted monarch toward the billions of cells, bacteria, and viruses that comprise us, rather than like a harsh ruler. As you can see, the subject's intricacy necessitates consistent practice, tenacity, extensive research, and serious debate.

This is why I wanted a biohacking session at the World Changers Summit, and I requested Prof. Panfili to grant me the privilege of speaking about stem cells and regenerative medicine. I've known Adolfo Panfili for 40 years; he is not only my doctor but my friend and colleague.

I can only say that I've witnessed 40 years of continual scientific progress, devotion, and evolution. We did not always agree or take the same road, but we always appreciated and assisted one other from our diverse perspectives. I continue to find in him the support, stimulus, and evolutionary progress that I desire for everyone. Prof. Panfili possesses a collaborative spirit, as well as a curiosity and boldness that the scientific and, especially, medical communities require. Bureaucracy, protocols, restrictions, dogmas, and anxieties frequently kill more than mistakes. In fact, I believe that ethics and bravery, rather than fear or petty economic interests, should guide us into the future.

Today we have come together to reflect on the text and information provided by Prof. Panfili, knowledge whose origins I am aware of and which, for me, represents the illuminated path of a cohesive and happy existence. Please, enjoy this enthralling reading.

Chapter 1

The Only Handbook of Orthomolecular Biohacking (OB)

One dervish said, «One day I finally decided to set out on the path. However, I did not know how to proceed. It is strange: it was a dog who suggested it to me.
He had stopped in front of a puddle and his figure was reflected in the water. Immediately I noticed that he was afraid and would not stop contemplating his image. In fact, he thought another dog was threatening him.
That's why he didn't move, for fear of being attacked. But then, finally, he overcame his hesitation and threw himself into the puddle. It was then, that, as if by magic, the other dog vanished, leaving him master of the field. Can you now understand me, if I tell you that it was a dog that showed me the Way?»
Joannes Yrpekh
(from «The Way of Maat. Lights on Ancient Egyptian Wisdom.»)

By expanding the quality and duration of life, man needs inside/outside regeneration from the inside out, that is, total regeneration of his entire physical and spiritual being.
Reversing the hands of the biological clock is not simple, but possible. It is appropriate to keep in mind that regeneration is won only through the simultaneous exercise of will, intuition and reasoning. Through their complete concordance man is able to develop his faculties to incalculable levels. The soul possesses dormant peculiarities and sensitivities that initiation awakens. **With Kaizen (from Japanese for «change for the better continuous improvement») in-depth enthusiastic study and constant application man can bring himself into conscious relationship with the occult forces of the universe.**
With prodigious effort, one can achieve direct spiritual perception (channeling) and open paths outside of space and time by making oneself capa-

ble of embarking on one's inner hero's journey to rediscover the Alchemical Elixir of regeneration and well-being that was thought to be lost.
Accept challenges even if at first they find you reluctant and recalcitrant to change. Threshold keepers will try to dissuade you, making a thousand excuses, but do not desist and smile at them in return and continue undaunted in the search for your inner grail.

Fear not because mentors and fellow travelers will flock to enlighten your path. Do not give up now or ever. Once you overcome your fears and insecurities, you can rise to the surface richer and different than before.

Only then will you realize that you have conquered fate and gained in this world the divine karmic awareness of the true self.

Only then can the initiate become initiator in turn, prophet and theurg, that is, seer and awakener of souls, for only he who commands himself can constructively interact with others, only he who is free can liberate and finally become the commander of his own soul and the captain of his life.

The first Orthomolecular Biohacking exercise is to remove the semantic sabotage that inhibits cell regeneration, Osho (the Puna philosopher) asserted that **«the mind lies.»** And he was right.
Every time you blow an extra candle on your birthday, you are sabotaging your autopilot, because on a subconscious level, you have triggered a kind of final countdown, bringing you closer and closer to the time of the «final farewell.» If the average lifespan is 80.5 years for men and 84.8 for women, according to ISTAT 2023 data, turning one year older is not a kindness to our autonomic nervous system, which will do its best to fall within life expectancy (80/85 years).

Poet John Donne first and Ernest Hemingway later in 1940, said "For whom does the bell toll? Never ask for whom the bell tolls, it tolls for you." The clear reference to the moment of truth that describes the infinite moment of passing away underlies the concept: no man is independent of the rest of the world.

Each individual has established his or her own «unique mental filtering» system to process millions of bits of data that are absorbed through the senses. We are capable of triggering a series of actions, more or less consciously, that hinder the achievement of our long-term goals.

THE MOST COMMON CAUSES OF SSS (SELF SEMANTIC SABOTAGE)

- Fear of change and the unknown, resulting in a preference for the much-famous «comfort zone» and what we have always made statements such as: I can't do it, I don't have time, I don't have money, I'm too old, I'm too young, and all the plausible excuses in order to procrastinate.
- Performance anxiety: the need to achieve the goal: which causes us to somatize so much anxiety and worry, that if we somehow self-sabotage first it is better, so the anxiety drops and it will not be necessary to bring out excellent performance.
- Nikephobia, literally means «fear of winning» (Greek terminology composed of «*nike*» victory and «*phobos*» meaning fear). It is a phobia characteristic of the world of sportsmen, especially in the competitive field, but it can be found in any situation that life offers in terms of competition.
- Self-evaluation. We think we do not deserve something and then we self-sabotage ourselves with low self-esteem. Ultimately we set ourselves up for failure because we are intimately convinced that we do not deserve success, happiness, longevity, etc.
- We tend to see the glass as half empty instead of half full. We are used to boycotting ourselves, due to ancient psycho-social-familial conditioning and focus on failures: instead of focusing on all our victories by taking a destructive negative viewpoint feeding a vicious cycle of DE-EPOWERMENT.
- Further example: my parents also died young therefore I will die young...

The causal concatenation of Self Semantic Sabotage (SSS) often goes back a long time in our existence, the important thing is to become aware of it and to realize that self-sabotage can be defused. Exactly as 007 did when seconds before the explosion, he managed to defuse the device saving humanity.
This manual will help you, novice secret agents, to hack the system ethically and correctly, finally defusing

The device that you alone had initiated. Did you know that more than 96% of our impending fears will never occur? Therefore, it is better to be more epicurean and avoid literally «dying» from flimsy fears.
Whenever we think about change we want everything as soon as possible. We should not be in a hurry, because small steps make big paths, and it is these metamorphic changes that matter most.

Chapter 2
OB: Orthomolecular Biohacking

«I think every person should enjoy life. Figure out what you enjoy doing and look for a job where you have skills and can continue to experience that kind of satisfaction.»

Linus Pauling

OB (orthomolecular biohacking) is a multi-facted mode to expand the performance of the your health, achieve and maintain and enlarge your goals. Biohacking is an extremely compact and efficacious biological approach to bring together all the arrows in the quiver of well-being and quality of life available to human beings, with a distinct ecological impact to the preservation of the person and the environment. Skillfully blending supplements such as amino acids, vitamins, minerals, cryotherapy, advanced training techniques, inductive sleep techniques with reactivation of dopaminergic circuits, mindset expansion, and, to acquire and maintain this positive bio enthusiastic charge, therapy radiant (RLT) with red light.

To incorporate a mindset of abundance is to realize positive and lasting changes.

Do you need help incorporating biohacking into your life? Talk to a professional, become a coach and start educating yourself on the subject. Once you are ready, your body will thank you. This book is a thank you to the Universe from a very lucky man who was karmically given the opportunity to choose a fascinating and generous incarnation. That is why I asked for and was granted in identifying a family that would guarantee to match humanism and science at the same time.

From an early age, I was fortunate to have been educated by a Mother, an excellent writer and teacher, in the unconditional expression of joy, happiness and enthusiasm in the activities I was doing. On Father's side I was able to secure, as a first-rate element, a man with great spirituality, idealistic to a fault, inclined to Eastern doctrines. An excellent lawyer, my father had fought as a volunteer on the Slavic front in World War II and then retired for ten years to India and meditated...

Sharing has always been my empathic mode of aggregation, the convergence of many lives at the center of a wheel represented by the enthusiasm and motivation to live to fufill of one's possibilities.

IMPROVE LIFE PERFORMANCE

This is not an expansionist narcissistic delusion of omnipotence, so much as a desire to want to maximize personal energy resources with the practicality of a shareable text that essentially helps others live better. Narcissism becomes pathological when oblative capacity (from the Latin *oblativus*: given, spontaneously offered) is lacking. A handbook to help identify future paths and ambitions by grasping essential data such as one's genetic background history, which, if properly interpreted, can provide valuable information.

To achieve a goal, we cannot disregard following a precise course and then directing the sails according to the prevailing winds. No pursuit of institutional acclaim, but rather a desire to pursue tangible results and goals to paradigm through unstructured creative free thinking (*ground evidence*).

What it would be like to develop through this reading creative lateral thinking by integrating it with the monocratic and crystallized linear thinking foraged by multinational corporations aimed only at economic profit and certainly not at protecting the health of humanity. The goal is to awaken through a careful analysis of events outside the stigmas of rotogravure pseudoscience and power-peddling journalism.

It has been fun to range in the various fields of knowledge, from robotics, to chemistry-metabolics, to quantum physics, to insights in the area of philosophies and religions. The study of psychology and sociology were very helpful in amplifying the multidisciplinary approach.

An important influence was my meeting with Professor Linus Pauling, double Nobel laureate in Chemistry and Peace, who transmitted to me the

rigor of the scientific approach integrated with the thought creative lateral and Ted Morter Jr, one of the greatest chiropractors who ever lived, who passed on to me all levels of BEST Chiropractic, which I have been using successfully for more than 30 years.
Why talk about Biohacking at a time when we are witnessing the most important transition ever observed in recent centuries? At this time we need to seize the infinite possibilities and opportunities that the global transition proposes. The selection of the environment, manipulated by man, poses the need to know ourselves better, paraphrasing the likes of Socrates, Hippocrates and Aristotle. On the pediment of the Delphic oracle and in my soul is enscribed with the fire of curiosity in large letters the imperative aphorism: «NOSCI TE IPSUM,» or know thyself. How many times have you reached the end of the day or week realizing that you have been running after urgent mtters sacrificing time to devote to the things that are really important to you, your business or family?

Come to think of it, time is the same for everyone, in that there are no people who possess it, only individuals who know how to organize it better by devoting it to things that improve the quality of life itself. What else is possible? How could it be better than that?

Your time is the same as that used by Jesus of Nazareth, Buddha, Mother Teresa of Calcutta or Gandhi. We are confident that you too can achieve splendid results. There are no shortcuts or alternative systems, no magic pills or miracle diets. You are the real living miracle. Let your enthusiasm be the inexhaustible fuel of your success. With the right dopaminergic motivation, you can climb Mount Everest (everyone can reach its metaphorical summit if they really want to), whereas without enthusiasm, sometimes you would not even go downstairs to buy the newspaper.

Time, Enthusiasm and Creativity are an inseparable, precious and invaluable **trinomial**, everyone naturally receives a fair amount of them as a dowry, so manage them well, do not waste them and, most importantly, do not allow anyone to rob you of them. Beware of time and enthusiasm thieves, often masked by bad habits and routines that obscure the urgency and importance of real priorities.
Each of us stands *«on the heart of the earth, pierced by a sunbeam and it is immediately evening.»* Each is still and motionless only in the illusion of being.

You are special, unique and unrepeatable beings, and you will succeed. Decide on change, here and now! My most genuine aspiration is to outline with you essential and precise hypotheses for increasing individual performance, summarized in an agile and quick program that provides tangible results. For example, the use of a good supplement based on amino acids, vitamins and minerals to be taken a couple of times a day in concomitance with a healthy physical activity, without becoming hostages to nerve-wracking and interminable workouts in the gym, could greatly reduce the stress that accompanies daily life and enable you to achieve greater results and, more importantly, greater success and satisfaction. You could, but have you thought to check first whether your gut is able to appreciate and receive all these gifts?
Forty years ago I was the first in Europe to talk about supplements, amino acids, beginning to «hack» the biochemical individuality possibly improving it. With today's awareness, it is finally possible to improve assimilative capabilities first by rebalancing the gut microbiome setup. Imagine the digestive system as a large apartment building, where, before sending Christmas presents, it is good to check that there is someone in the house otherwise one would run the risk of unnecessarily wasting huge resources.

Onward, then, full steam ahead!
Biohack yourself!

Chapter 3

I want to be an Orthomolecular Biohacker.

Check the inside/outside biology of life

«The greatest discovery of my generation.
Is that man can change his life simply by changing his mental attitude.»

William James

The Science does not have the answers in its pocket for every question. Until now we have structured our «growth» on Outside Biology instead of mastering our internal Biology. Cosmetic surgery helps all right, but sometimes it produces wonderful morphologically unimpeachable containers, which, however, do not express the quality of an **«inner health.»** Shortcuts that do not lead far. The Greeks spoke of this kind of beauty, ***kalokagathia***, or the ideal of physical and moral perfection. At this point how can we not refer to the archetype of the first Biohacker who on his skin experienced the courage of his own ideas? I am talking about my teacher, Professor Linus Pauling (read about it in the chapter on Peace in this text).
I consider myself rightly or wrongly a poor clone.
Pauling's ingenious insight into the metaphor inherent in Biohacking, which implies taking control of one's biology by making changes to one's lifestyle, diet or even one's body to improve health, performance or *well being,* by disregarding the mainstream and the static and obscurantist thinking connected only to the drug. The Biohacker opposes the divine presumption to control everyone's life through the mechanical sprinkling of cheap chemical molecules. Reviewing Professor Linus Pauling's as-

tounding scientific and social curriculum, one cannot help but notice that he published thousands of pages on the use of vitamin C to cure a virus such as the Common cold... yet despite the two Nobel prizes he received for his studies in the field of chemistry, they were to no avail, as they failed to prevent him from criticism by the pharmaceutical lobbying pseudo inquisition of the time 55s-50s, which discriminated against his documentary achievements to the point of not granting him a passport to go to Sweden to discuss the award of his possible third Nobel Prize for his studies on the DNA double helix.

Pauling, revealing himself a man of courage and determination, supported by his wife Ava Helen Miller, **is in effect the Founding Father of this modern science of Biohacking**.

Defending one's own welfare and that of humanity are the primary ways that science must not and cannot ever forget.

It is also (but not only) about using science and technology in a do-it-your-self way to «hack» the body's biology without necessarily delegating control of one's free genomic individuality to others. In a near-future reality it will be possible to fly as high as Icarus by manipulating to one's liking with AI even one's own DNA amino acid sequences.

Neither more nor less so as has already been done with body art, tattoos, piercings, etc. The piracy of the Tortuga brothers will return to plow the digital seas of the relatively unexplored ocean of genetics.

This handbook aims to draw up orthomolecular guidelines certainly not to harness biohackers, but to ensure their survival and expand their potential in a new suburban nihilistic culture that will seek to engulf them as heterogeneous examples of diversity «OUT OF THE BOX»...

Science is doubt itself in that it will never confer on us an absolute and indisputable schism, especially about the most recent happenings.

Science is not stuffed with exclamation points, but is redolent with many question marks in sharp break with the claim to produce a perfect, prepackaged answer to every question.

If science were a bartender, it would be a wonderful cocktail of truth, uncertainty, and enthusiastic childlike wonder, elements necessary to always find a balance.

Somewhat like Newton who perceived himself as a child on the seashore playing with seashells, aware that *«the great ocean of truth stretched out before him to be discovered»,* the Biohacker is a kind of Newton exhumed from the ashes of a Phoenix, a metaphor for a science in its twilight years that through them must be reborn with challenges, uncertainties and creativity, stronger and crisper than before. Apodictic extremes in which technology is seen in a dualistic way, as a new deity or as infernal drift.
Biohacking is not just what you read on Wikipedia, but as you will learn from reading this manual, much, much more...

Chapter 4

The biohacker practices the *kalokagathia*

«Sometimes from one spark a fire breaks out.»
Lucretius Caro - De rerum natura

In the Greek culture of the fifth century B.C.E., the KALOKAGATHIA represented the ideal of man's physical and moral perfection. To better understand why the Greeks represented the progenitors of modern Biohackers we have to consider the etymology of this intriguing word; in fact, the word comes from the crasis of *kalosis*, which means beautiful in Greek, and *atos*, which means good. Literally it coincided with the identity of what is beautiful and what is good both from an objectively material point of view and in the realm of ideas of Platonian memory. The term of beautiful and good was often understood as valiant in war and as possessing all the virtues somewhat as we might imagine the modern Biohacker, who harbors in himself the expertise, the knowledge of the man of science and the sensitivity of the physician and healer at the same time. We are talking about a beauty connected to moral behavior; going back in time we might find that this concept might spring from a Homeric legacy introduced in Athens beginning in the second half of the fifth century B.C. by the Sophists, who condensed by this dominant intellectual expression in the oratorical and political career without referring to any military aspect, but rather to a moral value of virtue and justice. Finally, Plato posits of *kalokagathia* an aristocratic ideal that distinguishes the wise man from the masses: one who devotes himself to scientific research or some other intense intellectual activity must also devote himself to the body and its movement, practicing gymnastics, while one who devotes himself with care to shaping the body must provide in compensation for the soul its movements, resorting to music and everything related to philosophy if he wants to be rightly called both beautiful and good. In conclusion, in the genesis of the modern Biohacker, *kalokagathia* should be the object of the his education to excellence since all good and beautiful qualities must be kept in practice as much as wisdom. Beauty connected with action is complementary to the beautiful and good, in short what is beautiful cannot but be good and what is good is necessarily beautiful.

OPERATIONAL MODES OF BIOHACKING

Cold immersion practices and use of ice baths. The use of heat therapy and saunas.

The use of smartwatches and other formative feedback tools. Whole body vibration therapy.

Pulsed electromagnetic field therapy (PEMF). Red light therapy (RLT) for healing and recovery.

For the more secular hackers, instead, begin seeking out «escape channels» sometimes creatively, sometimes in seemingly disrespectful ways (toward stances raised on the altars of truth) of rigid and stale patterns in order, if necessary, to break static crystallized rules that have formed beliefs and habits in most people. In spite of self-styled prophets, ***biohacking is the process of implementing smart tips (wise advice) to intervene in lifestyle quality «scientifically guided» and not necessarily in the garage at home on a Sunday afternoon...***
To increase optimal performance throughout the journey of a human being's existence who wishes to change his or her views and reasonably wonders how it can be better than that and what else is possible? Biohacking is not a burst of Asprey-like narcissistic contemplation celebrating one's choices as fundamental standards to be imposed on anyone, but rather an invitation to descend into the deep labyrinth of the self to discover your own true and unique alchemy of your Biohacker's journey, finding your true existential *mission*.

One of the most inspiring and motivating projects of the OM approach is to create a database from individual experimenters and researchers in order to interpret them by expanding them through evaluation with an artificial intelligence-based algorithm that will make multiple and endless ways to live better plausible and available.

Certainly, the figure of the physician as we understood it will also be reshaped, not in the sense that it will necessarily have to disappear, but that it will be supplemented by operational emergency physicians led by the hand by their own voice assistant.

It is a very broad term that encompasses a wide range of actions, all with a similar goal: optimizing health. Commonly referred to as «do-it-yourself» biology, biohacking often involves self-experimentation to gather ultra-personalized data and feedback.

Take sleep as an example: the importance of sleep is based on sound science; it serves as an organic regenerative moment. Through it, the organism is reborn N times, recovers, repairs and replenishes essential hormones. Quality sleep is linked to a robust immune system and healthy aging. In contrast, poor sleep can lead to various health problems, including a weakened immune system, a shorter lifespan, and an increased risk of obesity, type II diabetes, and cardiovascular disease. Optimizing sleep has become a primary goal for the biohacker. With new technologies and wearable devices such as Oura Ring, Whoop, and Fitbit, you can now easily monitor and use sleep data to improve it: biohacking is all about collecting data through AI. Science requires us to get out of the «coercion to repeat» and pull our heads out of the stagnant water of habits and preconceptions to finally draw a big, invigorating, regenerating breath at the top of our lungs.

Alarmist assertions that paint Hackers as dangerous exalted visionaries of our present time coming through a time gap from the barricades of distant 1968 to launch «Matrix Tricks» instead of red-hot Molotov cocktails to shatter the current unstable certainties dictated by fear and marketing lobbies do not hold up.

Will today's Heracles, the Biohacker, defeat the Hydra of Lerma?

A nine-headed snake that figuratively represents any evil that is seriously detrimental to society and by its very strength and spread is difficult to eradicate.

Some "conspiracy-minded well-wishers" propose hackers as visionaries pursuing ultra-narcissistic visions of the body understood as NFT of artworks from the founding groups of body art.

Nothing could be more false.

From the hackers the orthomolecular approach from Panfili to Pauling is transposed the spirit of indomitable experimentation and speculative inquiry that in the 1970s paved the way for a series of exceptional discoveries made by other (sometimes very young) hackers who were able, with few and rudimentary means, to pursue innovative projects and to «force» more and more of the capabilities of the machines then available.
When the interest of hackers began to show a drift towards hardware as well it was thus that a new need arose: that of spreading computers to the masses, essentially creating the spark of a new cybernetic relationship between man and machine as long as we confront the brilliant innovation of AI (artificial intelligence) today.
Just as Body Art induces and seduces with the theme of corporeality related to an unusual use of the body: aesthetic events are positioned as a moment of deep investigation of the self, and corporeality is established as the privileged territory of identity research.
All this on second thought could be a thorn in the side of politicians, economists and lobbyists who are unlikely to be able to control those who emerge from the masses and curiously raise their heads above the herd...
Interestingly, both of these movements: Body Art and Biohackers were born within the processes of historical and social change closely linked to the events of the late 1960s and early 1970s.

Biohackers are people and communities doing biological research in the hacker style, that is, outside of institutions, in an open and lateral form to use a term dear to De Bono, sharing information. They are experiences in which, through networking or by building labs that anyone can access and participate in, they try to make biology more collective and open.
Just as happens in the production of open source software.

Altering one's genetic constitution is increasingly becoming a consistent excision in a mainstream that increases neuro-sedation with repetitive mantras typical of monocratic and crystallized linear thinking, such as «you can't do it, no one has ever done it, it's impossible it's not the right time, it's dangerous»... if you don't challenge the impossible you can't achieve the possible the first hacker on the street corner would answer you...

Intriguing, no longer visionary, the possibility of opening the black box of life in defiance of beliefs and religions, stealing like Prometheus the Sacred Fire from the gods. Was it permissible to use CRISPR-like genetic modification tools with a technique using the CAS9 molecule and a bacterial system found in about half of bacteria and 90 percent of archaebacteria?

The number of technical possibilities available to man increasingly raises the question of the relationship that must exist between technical possibility and the possibility or moral permissibility of applying these same techniques. This manual was created to create a real balance between aspirations and opportunities that this magical future is lavishly unfolding to us.

Let's take advantage of it! No guillotine for the brave and courageous Biohackers!

Chapter 5

Linus Pauling and Peace

The scientist who tried to save the world

«Let us try to live in peace, whatever our origin, our faith, the color of our skin, our language and our traditions. Let us learn to tolerate and appreciate differences. Let us strongly reject all forms of violence, of oppression, the worst of which is war.»

Margaret Hack

Why a chapter dedicated to Peace? Why not! It is not off-topic, without Peace humanity will never be in balance, it is essential to understand that Orthomolecular Biohacking is a path where every part of our living needs harmony and beauty. And it is in universal peace that it finds its roots. Linus Pauling gave ample evidence of this.

LINUS PAULING, A VISIONARY AND A SCIENTIST

I receved numerous lessons from Pauling, all invaluable, and many shared through my many texts on Orthomolecular Biohacking.

Of his prolific and unstoppable streak as a Science storyteller, one sentence in particular has marked me outside disquisitions on chemistry, physics and covalent bonds: *«If you want to change your destiny, you must have the courage to dare.»*

How many of us are ready to truly seize the moment?

«Carpe diem» stated Horace, and he was right! With the small addition of trusting as little as possible in tomorrow.

The train of happiness passes only once in a lifetime and makes no stops, if you do not have the courage to jump on at the drop of a hat you will have to be content to live with what you have for fear of daring.

Seize this divine inspirational spark to run and jump on top of that train that leads to discovering new, different and unexpected places, emotions and worlds that can change the kaleidoscopic «sliding doors» of your life.

To grasp the meaning of what I am saying follow me in this simple reasoning based on lateral thinking: if the morning before operating on ten heart transplant patients the heart surgeon woke up completely drunk it would probably be carnage.

The harm caused by the drunk surgeon's behavior would not be limited only to the poor unfortunate ten patients. The consequences would also extend to the offspring that will never be born (children, grandchildren, great-grandchildren by these never born) because of the drunken surgeon's unintended act; now, since it is statistically believed that the average man will encounter

10,000 people in your life, try to do the math. Of course that's a lot of people, but if each of you changed the lives of only ten of those people and each of those people changed the lives of ten other people-just ten-what would happen? Then in five generations - 125 years - the graduating class of my class in 2023 will have changed the lives of eight hundred million people.

Eight hundred million people-think about it! - more than twice the population of the United States. Isn't that incredible?

Let's take the statistical projection one step further and let another generation pass and you will see the entire population of the world, or eight billion people, change. So what are you waiting for to throw the pebble into the wishing pond as well?

Pauling made me realize that Science as well as social activism are needed outside of politics to ensure a future worth living not only for ourselves, but especially for our descendants.

Pauling's real and unquenchable treasure, besides the various Nobel Awards he received, was to have cultivated within himself that wonderful «CHILD-LIKE WONDER» that made his life designing and inspiring.

We all remained positively contaminated in one way or another by Pauling's awe and entering into a working relationship with him has been the key to many existences. To fully grasp his attitude as a scientist and activist I recommend reading his text «NO MORE WAR» which warns about the essential concept of choosing the right train. Have you ever wondered how important it is to «choose»?

How will your decisions today affect the choices of all your future descendants in the unstoppable flow of life?

Be careful about boarding a train that will end up on a dead end track at some point along the way, but once you get on board believe it!

Peace is the opposite of war, with one big difference: to achieve peace requires the goodwill and commitment of all; while to wage war it is enough for only one person to desire it. For peace to exist in the world, everyone's commitment is needed.

THE IMPORTANCE OF A SOCIAL CONSCIENCE TO OPPOSE WARS

«I believe that only one thing makes the realization of a dream impossible: the fear of failure.»
Paulo Coelho

Where have the barricades of '68 gone, where are our aspirations and ideals, our promises our social commitment hidden? The experiences of Mahatma Gandhi in India, Martin Luther King and Linus Pauling in the United States, and Nelson Mandela in South Africa, marked milestones in the history of «nonviolent revolutions» for social transformation and the pursuit of Peace. Now all of a sudden these «beacons in the night» of Humanity who sacrificed their lives for the absolute ideal of Peace are being extinguished by winds of war and mass genocide. Just think that today's politicians were the young people who chanted slogans such as «Make love and not war» in peace marches in the 1970s. Schizophrenia of the masses, could one argue inspired by Gustav Le Bon (Psychology of Crowds - 1895)? Where have those trampled and forgotten ideals gone in our days, where everyone is ready to fight his own war against his neighbor to protect his own little garden?
Peace is the basis of civil coexistence among people. There, where Peace is lacking, people suffer, but the ones who pay the highest price of long and unnecessary wars are always and especially the children, who are robbed of their future and denied any planning for life.

Pauling argued that there are no just wars even though for theologians and philosophers of many religions war would even be considered just in at least three cases:

Defensive if declared to right a wrong suffered.

To **reset** the effects of a previous conflict.

Punitive if conducted to punish those who had caused serious harm. In any case it was to be fought in moderation, in a proportionate manner.

After the horrors of Hiroshima and Nagasaki in August 1945, a distraught Einstein said, **«I have no idea what weapons will be needed to fight World War III, but the fourth will be fought with sticks and stones. In any case, if I had known, I would have been a watchmaker.»**
Peace is not just the opposite of war, Peace is not just the time space between two wars... Peace is more, it is the Law of Life itself.

Peace is when we act justly and when justice reigns among every single being. As long as man exploits man, as long as humanity is divided into masters and servants, there will be neither normality nor peace. Peace can last only where human rights are respected, where people do not go hungry, and where individuals and nations are free.

PAULING AND HIS STAND AGAINST NUCLEAR WEAPONS

«No Nuke, the Thousand and One Slags.»
Anonymous

During the 1950s Pauling and his wife became famous to the public through their crusade to stop atmospheric testing with nuclear weapons. In 1958 they submitted a call for a test ban to the United Nations in the form of a document signed by 9,235 scientists from 44 countries. Pauling's sentiments were also promulgated through his book «NO MORE WAR» («Never Again!» - 1958), this text contains an impassioned analysis of the implications of nuclear war for humanity.

Each nuclear device test spreads an additional load of radioactive elements to every part of the world. Each additional amount of radiation causes cascading damage to the health of human beings around the world and massive damage to the human germline such that it will lead to an increase in the number of children with severe neonatal diseases being born in future generations. The oxidation induced by these thoughtlessly performed tests increases the stress on the individual immune system while also increasing the rate of cancer occurrence.

As long as these weapons are in the hands of only three powers, an agreement for their control is feasible,» Prof. Linus Pauling wrote at the time **in a petition signed by more than 11,000 scientists from around the world and submitted to the U.N. Secretary-General**.

Pauling's petition was just one of many initiatives in a long list of activities he led against the nuclear arms race.

He stands head and shoulders above others, having being awarded (without sharing the prize with others) two nobel prizes in different fields. His path was rewarded, but even before that Pauling was a major figure in the scientific community, and he is still considered one of the greatest chemists of the 20th century.

In 1960 Pauling was called upon to defend his actions regarding the testing ban before a congressional subcommittee. By refusing to reveal the names of those who had helped him gather signatures, he risked going to jail, a stance initially condemned but later widely admired by the world. His work for world peace was recognized with the 1962 Nobel Peace Prize, awarded on October 10, 1963, the date the Nuclear Test Ban Treaty went into effect.

Pauling's Peace Prize aroused such antagonism from Caltech administrators that he left the institute in 1963. He became a staff member of the Center for the Study of Democratic Institutions in Santa Barbara, California, where his humanitarian work was encouraged. Although he was able to develop a new model of the atomic nucleus while working at the Center, his desire to do more experimental research led him to become a research professor at the University of California at San Diego in 1967. There he published a paper on the theory of orthomolecular psychiatry with Prof. Abram Hoffer that explained how mental health could be achieved by manipulating substances normally present in the body. Two years later he accepted a position at Stanford University, where he worked until 1972.

PAULING AND VITAMIN C

Years later, while at San Diego and Stanford, Pauling's scientific interests focused on a particular molecule: ascorbic acid (vitamin C). After reviewing published reports on this vitamin he concluded that, if taken in sufficiently large amounts (megadoses), it could help fight major viral (colds, etc.) and other diseases.

The result of his fantastic research was the publication of the book ***Vitamin C and the Common Cold*** (1970), which became a best-seller. Pauling's interest in vitamin C in particular and orthomolecular medicine in general led him, in 1973, to found an institute that eventually bore his name: the Linus Pauling Institute of Science and Medicine. During his tenure at this

institute, he became embroiled in controversy over the relative benefits and risks of ingesting megadoses of various vitamins. The controversy intensified when he argued for the usefulness of vitamin C in the treatment of cancer. Pauling and his collaborator, Scottish physician Ewan Cameron, published their views in Cancer and Vitamin C supported by a myriad of paradigm clinical cases (1979). Also of note by the same authors ***Vitamin C and cancer***, a text dense with detailed studies and embarrassingly large clinical cases.
Their ideas were screened by funded experimental animal studies from the institute. Although these studies supported their ideas, investigations at the Mayo Clinic involving cancer patients did not corroborate Pauling's findings, who in any case did not have access to the setting of the materials and methods of the work in progress at the prestigious university.
Although he continued to receive recognition for his early achievements, Pauling's later work provoked considerable skepticism and controversy. His cluster model of the atomic nucleus was rejected by physicists, his interpretation of newly discovered quasi-crystals received little support, and his ideas on vitamin C were rejected by the medical establishment. In an attempt to raise funds to support his increasingly struggling institute, Pauling published ***How to Live Longer and Feel Better*** (1986), but the book failed to become the success he and his collaborators had anticipated.
Both Pauling and his wife developed cancer. Ava Helen Pauling died of stomach cancer in 1981. Ten years later Pauling discovered he had prostate cancer. Although he underwent surgery and other treatments, the cancer eventually spread to his liver.
He died on his ranch on the Big Sur coast of California.

Chapter 6

Physiology of meditation and mindfulness

«One grateful thought raised to heaven is the most perfect prayer.»
Lessing - Barnhelm's Minna

To live the healthiest life, you need a daily dose of positivity that flows precisely from an alkaline body. Instead of investing in stocks and watering with the anxiety of anticipation the little garden of investment, devote time to the wealth of the soul by meditating. More and more often you meet business captains, managers, secretaries of party, men of temporal power who surprisingly return in search of the roots of their inwardness, as if to transcend the illusory affabulation of money, the result of a convention with a Faust always ready in the shadows to snatch tired souls.
An ancient Zen koan tells of a man searching for the true Master who could enlighten him about the eternal secret of Life, and it just so happens that the pupil comes before a wise monk just as the latter was pouring himself some tea. Now you should know that tea for the Orientals is not a casual socio-gastronomic event, as Westerners understand it, but so much more. They devote themselves to this seemingly trivial customary gesture, an actual ceremony, otherwise known as: «Tea Ceremony.» That being the case, the young man in question began to subserve the old bard with a tirade about his own exploits, while the sage continued undaunted to pour the steaming beverage until the liquid began to overflow from the cup.
The bold and stilted pupil added, «stop, don't you realize what you are doing?».
The elderly Master, continuing unabashed to stir the steaming liquid with his face furrowed with a thousand wrinkles, smiled and with eyes pervaded with light and serenity replied, «You cannot fill a cup that is already full!».

The all too explicit moral of the story suggests that it is impossible to learn anything when you are too «full of yourself,» and that in order to receive a new message it is essential to empty the container first.

Getting rid of old preconceptions, suspending judgments, removing the frenetic activity of the mind deluded by an invasive and narcissistic ego, is the «*conditio sine qua non*» for changing the angle of evaluation of the phenomenon we are observing. This is possible through meditation and mindful prayer, acts of profound inner power, achievable by anyone, which allow one to learn the most important lesson of one's life, for which we all have incarnated and which the Japanese wisely define with a single pregnant and incisive term: «Youku,» which simply means white space, or back-ground of an ink drawing, what in TM is otherwise identified in the Gap (emptiness), which is generated between one thought and another, be-tween the thought object and the thinker himself.

Many patients fail to heal precisely because their encroaching ego overpowers the slender flame of the true self, entangled in the coils of illusory personalities, which seem to denigrate the deep thaumaturgic yearnings that dwell within each one. **Pramandha maintained that inside every man there is a master slumbering waiting to awaken... let us** therefore listen to this occult tenant and not give in to the sibylline temptations of a culture that weans us with freeze-dried milk and pain medications to dull our true consciences. Many people forget or ignore, because they are obnubilated by fallacious and subversive media, that the key to all healing is synonymous with internal growth, which often transits through the emblematic gallows of bodily pain. Without going over some frightening customs worthy of Jacopone da Todi, it is appropriate to stop and reflect that Mother Nature does nothing accidentally, and it is no coincidence that she has endowed us with a set of over 3,000,000 pain receptors and just 280,000 sensitive endings for experiencing pleasure. This certainly does not imply that we should be born only to suffer, but that probably if we are allowed to relate to external reality with a greater perceptual capacity for pain, there must be a reason. In biology, according to Spencer, the fittest survive, i.e., the one who succeeds before the other in getting to safety in the face of danger, through a refined and evolved survival function that the experience of pain can represent, if properly interpreted and not overshadowed by the taking of a symptomatic drug: medication in critical cases can save lives. This is not only right but essential to remember. Consider a person presenting with an acute life emergency, such as that of shock - at such a juncture it would be criminal not to administer intravenous cortisone to save him or her, claiming instead to want to treat him or her with a hawthorn herbal tea or a Bach flower, because one might lose the patient. Let the right medium of Buddhism's morality therefore be a comfort to the enlightened physician, who in such cases should be able to draw from his global store of information serenely, without becoming a slave to one idea or current of thought so that it may be respect for the meaning of life. Let us learn to listen to the message that pain can bring to those who will hear it. Administering an antispasmodic drug for the onset of a seemingly trivial digestive colic could mask the symptoms of peritonitis caused by suppurative appendicitis. In this case, the ill- advised use of the drug will certainly have spared the sufferer some suffering, but certainly not his life. So are we really convinced that pain is then such a bad counselor?

Turning off the red light on the dashboard alerting us to the lack of oil in the engine is not exactly a kindness to our car... Remember that the drug aimed at the exclusive removal of the pain symptom hides in addition to the doctor's insecurity, a non-causal approach and the result of the initiative will inevitably be devoted to the disappointment of the final expectations of a fearful well-being. Without remediation of the root causes of disease, there is no true healing, but only a temporary castling, we might say in terms dear to chess players. That is, an evanescent and deceptive metamorphosis of symptoms, which does not coincide with the overall state of health that we can all pursue. Pain and disease have brought Heaven and Earth closer together, and without them they would have ignored each other. **Ramakrishna in this regard stated that: «disease is the price the soul pays for the occupation of the body, just as a tenant pays rent for the apartment he inhabits.»**

Doctors are ready to help them listen to you, in fact you can already see some colleagues timidly beginning to prescribe transcendental meditation (TM), which is statistically an effective and inexpensive prevention tool.

In the U.S., some insurance companies are beginning to offer discounts on the health policies of people who are able to prove that they meditate or pray regularly, since it has been proven that those who are regularly engaged in these activities spend 77 percent less than others on medical expenses such as specialist visits, consultations, diagnostic tests, drugs and hospitalizations, as well as being less prone to cardio-cerebrovascular disorders, degenerative diseases such as cancers, etc... All this is not to say that God has become a giant jukebox bestowing prebends and favors, and that prayers are coins to make it work, indeed sometimes it happens that the jukebox does not play the selected record, since healing is modulated by an energetic carrier aware of the ideal attack site to perform its functions in the best possible way. It is like entrusting an economic capital to invest in the hands of a wise and enlightened asset manager whom one trusts blindly to the point of saying, «well, this is my savings, you do it, I trust you!» In short, when one affirms at the end of prayer the fateful, «Thy will be done!» one is entrusting oneself to an inscrutable cosmic will, but one that is surely fair and in any case expedient, for prayer acts and there is no formula or optimal way to present it to which everyone indiscrimi-nately must conform.

A study conducted at Dartmouth-Hitchcock Medical Center (DHMC) in 1995 would confirm that the best survival rates among 232 patients operated on in cardiac wards were shown in those who drew comfort from faith and meditation. In contrast, nonbelievers had three times higher mortality rates than believers.
Faithful practitioners had a blood pressure value more than 5 mm Hg lower than others, even when smoking and other risk factors were statis-tically (considered).
The incidence of depression, psychosomatic illness, prescription medication and illicit drug use, as well as suicide would be lower in TM believers and practitioners. Suicide rates are inferred to be four times higher among atheists than among those who attend masses regularly. Certainly a religious faith probably helps to better follow a diet that includes limiting food and alcohol abuse, drugs, etc., so the greater health would simply reflect healthier habits.
The mind is a television set with thousands of channels in order to see one distinctly, one must extinguish all the others.

Contemplating a mountain of snow, we are that mountain. Watching a noisy movie, we are that noisy movie. The channel we select is the channel we choose to be in that moment through the synergy of body, mind and soul.

When we turn on anger, we are anger. On the other hand, when we turn on peace and joy, we are peace and joy.

Focusing attention on a monotonous mantric-type sound or a single mandala-type image or specially selected sacred images induces a series of alkalizing physiological adaptations that are the exact opposite of the "fight or flight" response typical of the activation of the Orthosympathetic Nervous System, which produces great available energies in the span of a few moments, but at prohibitive metabolic costs because they are excessively acidifying.

With the practice of TM and mindful prayer (not mechanically repeated), the physiology of well-being is activated and objective benefits can be seen. In fact, heart rate, respiratory rate, brain waves slow down, muscles relax, and the effects of adrenaline and other stress hormones are finally alleviated. By routinely stimulating this response with relaxation, 75% of insomnia patients resumed a very regular sleep pattern, 35% of infertile women achieved pregnancy, and 34% of chronic pain sufferers reduced their in-take of painkillers.

In short, those who feel closer to God, Buddha, Manitou, Allah, etc., and make the most of it.

Feeling a strong inner presence is healthier and heals patients faster.

To combat the anxiety of separation that has been with us since we decided to inhabit the womb, we try to get in touch with God, and we do so through prayers that travel the same biochemical pathways as the response obtained through relaxation.

When you meditate you alkalize yourself by inactivating stress hormones: adrenaline, corticosteroids, etc., pursuing the lowering of Blood Pressure, slowing of heart rate and breathing rate, etc.

The mystical experience that TM and conscious prayer represent takes place in the same headquarters of the encephalon: the amygdala (small almond-sized anatomical formations that together with the hippocampus and hypothalamus constitute the limbic system (LS)).

The LS would turn out to be particularly involved with the complex sphere of spirituality of emotions and sexuality, through particular neuronal afferents that would mediate the release of the hormone melatonin secreted by the pineal gland related to the delicate functioning of the complex Immuno Neuro Psycho Endocrine System.

According to R. Joseph, a neurophysiologist at the Palo Alto VA Medical Center in California, stimulation of the LS (amygdala and hippocampus) would evoke visions of angels and demons in some subjects.

For example, chronic drug addicts have LS that are constantly bombarded with mystical stimuli, that in ancient times was only allowed to be achieved through bodily sacrifice, with exasperated asceticism, isolation, and special feeding and fasting techniques. Furthermore, pharmacological and neoplasm patients have a higher incidence of phobic-religious mania.

The epiphysis of subjects devoted to the constant and regular practice of TM for several years demonstrated excellent vascularization and overall less involutional fibrotic and senescence effects of the gland.

The ability to have religious and mystical experiences would present a neuro-anatomical and physiological basis related to changes in individual organic pH.

An alkaline pH would help in achieving those particular experiences of the high peaks by tuning the body more quickly to parasympathetic activity. The abolition of animal protein is warmly recommended in the unchallenged rules of many Cistercian monastic orders for finding God was intended to avoid the excessive acidification characterized by the defense-attack and flight-reactive reactions typical of the neurovegetative activation of the orthosympathetic system. Reducing the intake of protein and refined, and therefore acidifying substances ensures the replenishment of an adequate supply of alkaline reserve to activate those encephalic zones responsible for the establishment of the mystical experience itself.

WHO SAID MEDITATION IS NOT MEASURABLE?

Robert Miller in his book «Methods for Identifying and Measuring Healing Energies» (Doubleday & co, Inc., 1977) describes the development of an electromechanical transducer, already used at the U.S. Department of Agriculture by Kleuter and others, to measure the hourly growth of wild grass. The instrumentation consisted of a small device at lever connected with the growing end of the blade of grass to be measured. As the plant grew, the lever was raised and the mechanical displacement undergone by the medium was converted into a signal recorded on a strip of paper, which ran slowly underneath, like an electrocardiographic trace. The measuring system had been previously calibrated in the thousandths of an inch per hour range. Miller asked the Worral family if they would be willing to tune in at 9 p.m., their usual prayer time, visualizing the growth of blades of grass.

The unusual and disturbing aspect of the experiment was that the Worrals resided in Baltimore, which is more than 600 miles away from the laboratory site located in Atlanta, Georgia.

Before embarking on the evaluation, the device was turned on and previously calibrated for a few hours to make sure that the growth rate of the grass stems was stable.
The reading taken indicated a continuous and stabilized growth rate around values of 6.25 thousandths of an inch/hour. Miller hermetically sealed his laboratory to rule out the occurrence of any physical variation capable of affecting the experiment.
At exactly 9 p.m. as pre-arranged, the Worral family members began as planned to say their prayers, and the layout of the plants began to soar.
By the next morning, the track demonstrated an exceptional grass stem accretion of 52 thousandths of an inch/hour equal to a total increase of 840%.
The wonders of the experiment were not over, in fact after this period of time the growth of the grass slowed down significantly, though it never returned to its initial levels, remaining consistently higher than before the prayer therapy.
Even a Christian, a Buddhist, or a Hindu, when they pray or say a mantra or draw a mandala they are simply activating in the oldest and simplest of ways their capacity to self-alkalanize, and therefore to serve as a launching pad for their desires in the universe of their aspirations.
Later, when the Worral family was asked how they had achieved this prodigious effect, they replied that they had simply visualized the grass enveloped in golden light and energy.
At this point it is no longer convenient for anyone to be an atheist and it is convenient to start praying, consciously of course.
Today at the turn of this millennium we are crossing the threshold of a transitional phase in which humanity is converting mechanistic Newtonian-type ideas to the higher spiritual concepts that have led enlightened scientists such as Einstein, Tiller, Lorentz, to affirm «There is a God!»
The watershed between science and mysticism is now finally broken, the Berlin Wall has collapsed in the span of a very few years. The physicist and theologian contemplated the same star, but from two different vantage points, and now as never before they are and will be supportive of each other.

«The scientist studies the part of the tree that is above the ground, while the spiritual researcher studies the part that is below.»
Sai Baba

Chapter 7

Gurudev Sri Sri Shrankar the true biohacker of the spirit

If you have received the gift of Inner balance you must share it dedicating your full life to the fragiles : history of an everlasting friendship...

Adolfo Panfili, 2024

The multiple Nobel award prof Linus Pauling and Gurudev Sri Sri Shrankar influenced my life enormously. I've been really very lucky to have had the great opportunity to work with them side by side. Learning, inspiring, enlighting experiences that I have the pleasure to share with the all of you.

This is why I've decided to reserve to this very unique friends a paramount role in this revolutionary book of mine.

Isn't it amazing that also if they didn't know each other they were profoundly tuned on the same frequencies .

Many years ago I've met Gurudev Sri Sri Shrankar in Rome because he had orthopedic problems.

I gave him a full BEST Treatment that allowed him to recover immediately after a cervical/ lumbar block . After the successfull spine adjustment we started to talk and... becaming what today we can define: "good friends".

Today I'm proud to be their Diamond Medical Speaker all over the world because I trust from the deep of my hearth that Peace & Calm must be thought and spread up from north to south, from east to west in order to make a better world.

I really wish to share the main pillars of Gurudev's teachings:

1. Peace, he said, was neither lethargy, nor complacence, but inner balance and equipoise.
2. The Bhagavad Gita defined it as 'samatvamyogauchyate' (equanimity characterises yoga). As to dynamism in the world, which is the outer manifestation of the vitality of being.
3. Guruji suggested that it corresponds with another elucidation of yoga in the Gita, 'Yogahkarmasukaushalam' (yoga is skill in action).

4. Art of Living, he explained, was really the management of energy. When you are agitated or anxious, you lose perspective and efficiency. Better to be calm and purposeful.
5. Youth is full of energy and idealism, which are so necessary for our growth. Growth implies change, not stasis. In the eastern world this cor-responds to Eraclito's concept : "PANTA REI" from the Ancient Greek language means : "everything flows... And we must be part of the flow..."
6. Like trade and technology, traditions and textbooks also need constant renovation and revision, Guruji said.

The Art of Living Foundation

https://www.bangaloreashram.org/

The Art of Living is a form of Orthomokecujar Biohacking aimed to pursue the right self-direction for everyone in the unifying perspective of good living. The Art of Living aims to awaken in everyone the best ways for self-realization through a mix of modern and classic concepts, such as autonomy, authenticity and the "good life".

Is a volunteer-based, humanitarian and educational non-governmental organization (NGO).[1] It was founded in 1981 by Ravi Shankar.[2] The Art of Living Foundation has centers in 180 countries.

Pauling and Gurudev: both deeply spiritual beings not bound by inhibiting and restrictive thoughts, but rather in constant dynamic wonder at life and its mysteries.
Both united by the search for a dynamic and profound peace outside of religions and politics...
In summary I have collected some points in this chapter that I am sure will best illustrate their karmic similarities to you.

Religion is not just one, there are hundreds.
Spirituality is one.
Religion is for those who sleep.
Spirituality is for those who are awake.
Religion is for those who need someone to tell them what to do and want guidance.
Spirituality is for those who pay attention to their own inner voice.

Religion has a set of dogmatic rules.
Spirituality invites us to think about everything, to question everything.
Religion threatens and scares.
Spirituality gives inner peace.
Religion talks about sin and guilt.
Spirituality says: "learn from error".
Religion represses everything and in some cases is false.
Spirituality transcends everything, it brings you closer to your truth

Religion is about a god; he is not God.
Spirituality is everything and therefore it is in God.
Religion invents.
Spirituality finds.
Religion does not tolerate any questions.
Spirituality questions everything.

Religion is human, it is an organization with human rules.
Spirituality is Divine, without human rules.

Religion causes divisions.
Spirituality unites.
Religion seeks you so that you believe.
You have to seek Spirituality to believe.

Religion follows the precepts of a holy book.
Spirituality seeks the sacred in all books.

Religion feeds on fear.
Spirituality is nourished by trust and faith.

Religion lives in the lower astral.
Spirituality lives in Universal Consciousness.
Religion is about doing.
Spirituality has to do with Being.
Religion feeds the ego.
Spirituality pushes us to transcend.
Religion makes us renounce the world to follow a god.
Spirituality makes us live in God, without giving up on ourselves.
Religion is a cult.
Spirituality is meditation.

Religion fills us with dreams of glory in heaven.
Spirituality makes us experience glory and heaven here and now.
Religion lives in the past and the future.
Spirituality lives in the present.
Religion creates cloisters in our memory.
Spirituality frees our Conscience.
Religion makes us believe in eternal life.
Spirituality makes us aware of Eternal Life
Religion promises life after death.
Spirituality promises to find God within us during life and death.

We are not human beings having a spiritual experience. We are spiritual beings going through a spiritual experience, in a human body, in the making...

Chapter 8

Your true inspiration to change your judge

A million words cannot express what a glance can convey, and a million glances cannot express what a moment of silence can.

Sri Sri Ravi Shankar
(The Art of Living)

Gurudev Sri Sri Ravi Shankar is a global humanitarian, spiritual leader and ambassador of peace. Gurudev's vision of personal and social transformation through mental health and wellness has ignited a global movement in over 180 countries, uplifting the lives of more than 500 million people

Build upon your experience of freedom from the Happiness Program with a profound spiritual immersion. The Art of Living's Advance Meditation Program is a residential program that takes you deeper into your spiritual practices with advanced insights on the laws governing our mind and emotions as well as advanced breathing techniques that are easy to remember and can be practiced at home.
The hollow and empty meditations taught in the program along with other group processes bring about a deep cleansing from within leaving you feeling energetic and fresh for months on end.

KEY ASPECTS OF THE ADVANCED MEDITATION PROGRAM
Deep Meditation
A set of "Hollow and Empty" guided meditations created by Gurudev Sri Sri Ravi Shankar are the core part of the program. These meditations are geared towards drawing out the deepest layers of stress and tension from our nervous system.

Absolute Silence
Silence in the true sense is much more than not speaking. It is about giving a break to the chattering mind which gives way to renewing ourselves phy-

sically, mentally and spiritually. Silence during the program results in deeper rest to our mind, body and soul.

Mudras & Pranayama

Along with breathing exercises and advanced meditations, a series of simple and effective Pranayamas and Mudras - a subtle technique to balance the mind and emotions, are taught in the program which can be practiced along with other meditations.

Wisdom

Unite the body and mind with morning authentic forms of yoga and meditation to start a day. Explore the pillars of knowledge which open up multiple dimensions of our perceptions about various aspects of life, world around us and aspects of life beyond self.

Weekly Part II Program

The Art of Living International Center brings you the weekly part II program to give the much needed vacation you have been waiting for, both for your body and more importantly for your mind. The weekly part II programs happen every week at the Art of Living International Center

Chapter 9

OB: when stem cells make a difference

"Without stem cells we will no longer be here".
A. Panfili, 2024

Interview with Prof. Adolfo Panfili, Stem Cells World Leader

WHAT ARE STEM CELLS

The stem cells are immature cells that are not yet specialized, that is, cells that do not yet perform a specific function within the organism. At this particular stage of development
The cell has the ability to reproduce into other stem cells and generate specialized precursor cells that are destined to differentiate and transform into tissue and organ cells. This peculiarity of theirs makes it possible to provide the human organism with replacement and regeneration of cells in organs and tissues damaged due to physiological cell aging, disease or accidents. The stem cells most widely used for therapeutic purposes are embryonic stem cells and adult stem cells. The use of embryonic stem cells, for therapies or research, is at the center of a heated scientific-ethical debate. Although embryonic stem cells have a greater proliferative capacity and are totipotent, that is, capable of generating all types of cells, extracting them inevitably requires the killing of a human embryo, which is why their use is banned in many countries. No ethical problems exist, however, for stem cells obtained from umbilical cord blood. These are adult stem cells, i.e., derived from an already developed organism, whose task is to generate new cells intended for the growth, maintenance and repair of organs and tissues. These are multipotent cells, capable of transforming into certain specialized cell types. The adult stem cells contained in the blood of the umbilical cord are hematopoietic, meaning they can generate white blood cells, red blood cells and platelets on par with those in bone marrow. Therefore, umbilical cord stem cell transplantation is indicated to treat children and adults with all those diseases that require bone marrow transplantation.

STEM CELLS FROM UMBILICAL CORD BLOOD

Cord blood contains stem cells capable of curing serious diseases that cannot be treated with conventional drugs and therapies. These are a special type of stem cells, called hematopoietic stem cells, capable of efficaciously combating many hematological, immunological, genetic, metabolic and oncological diseases. Transplants of umbilical cord stem cells make it possible to successfully treat various forms of leukemias, lymphomas, anemias, myelomas, bone marrow aplasias, thalassemias, and some severe immune system defects. Therapeutic practices that are already widely established can go side by side with those that scientific research is developing with promising results. In the near future, it will be possible to have access to new therapies using stem cells to treat degenerative diseases such as Alzheimer's, Parkinson's disease, stroke, type 1 diabetes, muscular dystrophy, cardiovascular disease, and numerous other diseases for which there are no alternative treatments. Preserving umbilical cord stem cells for personal or family use is, therefore, an important preventive gesture now within everyone's reach. There is a growing awareness of how much hope for a cure is contained in umbilical cord blood, and more and more parents are deciding to safeguard this valuable health resource by storing stem cells for autologous use in private banks. Should the need arise, they will be immediately available, saving the patient a long, harried and sometimes fruitless search for a compatible donor, while averting the possibility of rejection or infection.

FROM THE DELIVERY ROOM TO THE CRYOPRESERVATION LABORATORY

The stem cell journey begins in the delivery room where, soon after the baby is born, umbilical cord blood is collected. The collection is painless and can be performed either by natural childbirth or by cesarean section, with no risk to either mother or infant. Thanks to the steady increase in the number of cord blood collections for autologous use, in Italy in 2008 there were about 10,000, the practice of this a simple procedure is now increasingly common, rapid, and safe. Once the collection is done, the cord blood sample is transferred to a special pressurized thermal container and shipped by dedicated courier to Bioscience Institute laboratories.
Sometime between 48 and 72 hours after delivery, the bag is submitted for analysis and started in the process of extracting the stem cells contained in the cord blood. Separated from other blood components, the stem cells are gradually brought to a temperature of -196°C and stored for twenty years in a nitrogen vapor cryobiology container. At the re-

quest of parents, a newborn screening for 60 metabolic diseases is also available free of charge. This test, carried out in the very first hours of life, makes it possible to detect the possible presence of diseases even before symptoms appear. By ascertaining the existence of a metabolic disease early and intervening with appropriate therapy, it can prevent serious damage to the body, especially neurological damage. Umbilical cord blood is collected immediately after birth and contains hematopoietic stem cells

WHAT TO DO TO PRESERVE UMBILICAL CORD STEM CELLS

Italian citizens are granted the right by the Ministry of Health to export and store, for preventive purposes, their children's cord blood in countries such as San Marino, where autologous storage is permitted. The procedure for obtaining export clearance from the Ministry must be submitted one month before the expected date of delivery. Bioscience Institute can, by calling the toll-free number 800 985 177, provide all information, forms and administrative support to easily complete the bureaucratic procedure. Also by contacting the toll-free number, or by filling out the online appli-cation form, it is possible to request shipment of the collection KIT, which must be delivered to the medical staff on the day of delivery.

Bioscience Institute staff also take care of Kit pickup and transport after delivery and, through its scientific committee, provide all medical information on therapeutic applications of stem cells and the current state of research. Bioscience Institute, in fact, in addition to cord blood preservation, carries out important scientific research activities on the use of stem cells in cardiology, orthopedics, surgery, and gynecology in collaboration with prestigious Italian and foreign universities, such as La Sapienza in Rome, the University of Bologna, the University of Urbino, UCLA in Los Angeles, and San Raffaele Hospital in Milan. In addition, Bioscience Institute collaborates steadily with INBB - Istituto Nazionale Biosistemi Biostructure (www.inbb.it), a consortium of more than 25 Italian universities that promotes and coordinates research and scientific and applied activities in the field of biotechnology. Citizens of the Republic of San Marino are not required to complete any bureaucratic procedures. To carry out cord blood storage, it is sufficient to deliver to the Bioscience Institute the report of HIV, TPHA, Anti-HTLV 1 and2, Hepatitis B and C tests, carried out in the last thirty days of gestation, and to request the Collection Kit.

AGING AND STEM CELLS

The dilemma of why we age is finally revealed. Aging depends on the number of stem cells in the body. At the time of birth we have about 200 stem cells for every 2 million cells, and at the age of 80, on the other hand, we have only one for every 2 million cells. The functionality of stem cells remains fairly stable during aging, although their numbers are significantly reduced during senescence. If we want to fight aging, we need to increase the amount of stem cells. Stem cells are capable of eclectic activities, including regeneration, revascularization, paracrine (hormonal reprogramming), and last but not least of all, anti-inflammatory action.

A HANDBOOK TO COMBAT AGING

Aging is a process that leads toward a generalized decline in the body's physiological functions. Contributing to this phenomenon are individual characteristics (genetics included) on which external factors such as lifestyle, diet and medication intake act. With this handbook we aim to share the most appropriate and mostly unknown, or even worse poorly understood, ways to increase individual performance capacity by improving lifestyles and using strategies condensed into a unique information in its field. This text is valuable because it gives us the right knowledge to live better and longer. As we have already stated, inflammation also plays a crucial role in the phenomena of aging; not surprisingly, it is a common feature of diseases associated with advancing age. There is even a specific term to refer to that form of chronic low-grade inflammation, not associated with infection, that develops with aging: inflammaging.

Inflammation is not an error of the body, but a weapon used by the body to fight against a wide variety of health threats, such as trauma, infection, stress, hydration, climate variations, etc. and more. In fact, there are forms of inflammation that are not triggered by microbes or injury. This type of inflammation can endanger health in a subtle way, without triggering obvious symptoms. Keeping inflammation levels below alert limits can help reduce risk factors for diseases associated with silent inflammatory phenomena. Genetic predisposition becomes eloquent when inflammation becomes rampant, bringing situations to the surface that would otherwise never have triggered conflict and disease.

Inflammation and oxidation go hand in hand, so it is no wonder that medically performed procedures involving strong oxidation can trigger inflammatory and aging processes (inflammaging), depression, degeneration, and cancer. Inflammation accompanies life at all stages and thus can be triggered by multiple types of noxious stimuli (microbes, viruses, parasites, trauma, nutrition, stress and damage to cellular structures, etc.). As life expectancy increases, the immune system faces all these stimuli for a long time. As a result, the inflammatory state can increase significantly, turning into what is called «chronic low-grade inflammation».

OB: BULLETS TO FIGHT INFLAMMATION

Targeted action on one's lifestyle can help reduce the stimuli that fuel the detected state of inflammation. Depending on the case, it might be useful to act, for example, on diet, or on stress levels. Taking dietary supplements with active ingredients that can modulate inflammation, always to be combined with an appropriate lifestyle, may also be helpful. Further investigations can help both to identify factors on which to act to reduce the inflammatory state, (e.g., microbiome analysis) and to assess the effects of the detected inflammation (particularly genomic instability analysis).

WHO TRIGGERS THE CHRONIC LOW-GRADE INFLAMMATION BOMB?

Inflammaging is triggered primarily by signals from within the body (hence termed «endogenous»), such as the presence of debris from cell death or oxidized or abnormally conformed proteins, which result in chronic activation of the immune system-a phenomenon that can be harmful. The factors that may contribute to its occurrence (damage to the body's macromolecules, metabolism, epigenetics, stress, protein balance, and stem cell activity) are interconnected and form an intricate web of elements capable of influencing each other, at the center of which is precisely inflammation.

Cellular and molecular mechanisms underlying inflammaging include:
The senescence of cells;
The malfunction of the mitochondria (the energy powerhouses of cells);
The malfunction of autophagy and degradation mechanisms in mitochondria;
the activation of the inflammasome (the complex intracellular multiprotein that identifies biological and nonbiological stressors);
The malfunction of the system that controls protein degradation;
The activation of the DNA damage response;
Alterations in the composition of the microbiota (so-called dysbiosis);
excess nutrients and overeating (i.e., eating too much food compared to the body's needs).

The latter can trigger a specific type of chronic inflammation called meta inflammation associated with metabolic disorders such as obesity and type 2 diabetes.
Chronic low-grade inflammation is associated neither with the classic symptoms of acute inflammation (swelling, pain, redness, and heat) nor with other symptoms or signs. Therefore, to detect its presence it is necessary to analyze the levels of molecules involved in inflammatory processes, such as cytokines and C-reactive protein (CRP).
It would be advisable to monitor a wide range of cytokines. For example, there are tests that evaluate more than 10. Of note is CYTOBALANCE from Bioscience, a leading global company in the field, which monitors 15 different markers of inflammation through a simple blood test. Detection of levels higher than those considered normal indicates the presence of an asymptomatic low-grade state of inflammation and the need to counteract it to protect one's health.

OB, CYTOKINE TESTING AND HEALTH STATUS

Proinflammatory cytokines are synthesized by cells of the immune system to regulate inflammatory responses. When they are produced for a limited period of time they exert a positive effect. When, however, their production is consistently high, as is the case with chronic low-grade inflammation, they can be harmful and promote the development of chronic diseases.
Some cytokines also regulate the production of PCR. The presence of this molecule is considered synonymous with inflammation. In fact, its levels are very low in healthy people, while they increase rapidly with inflammation. Not only that, PCR levels are associated with the development of inflammation-related diseases, such as cancers. Higher PCR concentrations, for example, are associated with higher risk of colorectal and breast cancer and lower survival to cancers of the esophagus, stomach, rectum, liver, pancreas, and ovary.

WHO TO RECOMMEND MY TESTS TO EVALUATE INFLAMMATION TO.

A true tailor-made program should be created for each patient to understand his or her metabolic, hormonal, and emotional universe. The monitoring of cytokine levels is useful and suitable for all those who wish to keep inflammation under control:

- during aging to combat inflammaging, the inflammation associated with advancing age
- In high-stress situations because stress is a major cause of inflammation

- When a healthy and balanced diet is not followed because malnutrition by excess and poor eating habits promote metabolic inflammation
- In case of exposure to proinflammatory molecules (hormones, smoking and other toxic substances can promote inflammation)
- In cases of intestinal dysbiosis (alterations in intestinal bacterial flora are associated with increased proinflammatory cytokines).

Chronic low-grade inflammation is a major cause of frailty and disease during aging. In fact, it is associated with health problems such as atherosclerosis, Alzheimer's disease, Parkinson's disease, type 2 diabetes, and cancers. In addition, it is one of the leading causes of death. Therefore, counteracting it can help both to live long and to do so in the best possible state of health.

Chapter 10

Orthomolecular Biohacking of the umbilical cord blood stem cells: a dream for the future of medicine

Umbilical cord blood collected at birth is a rich source of stem cells that can be used to treat diseases of the blood and immune system. Umbilical cord blood cells are taken from the umbilical cord (and placenta) after a baby is born, not from an embryo.

Unless donated, the placenta, umbilical cord, and stem cells they contain are discarded as medical waste.

Cord blood stem cells which have infinite medical potential are currently used in the treatment of several life-threatening diseases, and play an important role in the treatment of blood and immune system related genetic diseases, cancers, and blood disorders. Transplant recipients are less likely to reject a cord blood stem cell and DO NOT REQUIRE a perfect match as bone marrow transplants do.

Unless donated, the placenta, umbilical cord, and stem cells they contain are discarded as medical waste.

Transplantation of umbilical cord blood stem cells represents a major advantage in providing a new source of stem cells to patients in need. Private storage of cord blood stem cells clearly has value, in that it provides future patients and families with potential therapeutic options for transplant. Many recent studies showed that human umbilical cord blood stem cells have the potential to generate cells with neuronal characteristics. Therefore, the umbilical cord blood stem cells can be viewed as the stem cells source of choice for clinical and non-clinical research applications.

(S K Chakraborty et al. Mymensingh Med J. 2014 Jul. PubMed)

The umbilical cord blood is usually disposed of as an unwanted material after parturition; however, today, it is viewed as a regenerative medication so as to create the organ tissues. This cord blood gathered from the umbilical cord is made up of mesenchymal stem cells, hematopoietic stem cells, and multipotent non-hematopoietic stem cells having many therapeutic effects as these stem cells are utilized to treat malignancies, hematological ailments, inborn metabolic problem, and immune deficiencies. Presently, numerous clinical applications for human umbilical cord blood inferred stem cells, as stem cell treatment initiate new research. These cells are showing such a boon to stem cell treatment; it is nevertheless characteristic that the prospect of conservation of umbilical cord blood is gaining impetus. Current research works have demonstrated that about 80 diseases, including cancer, can be treated or relieved utilizing umbilical cord blood stem cells, and every year, many transplants have been effectively done around the world. However, in terms of factors, including patient selection, cell preparation, dosing, and delivery process, the treatment procedure for therapy with minimally manipulated stem cells can be patented. It is also worth thinking about how this patent could affect cord blood banks. Meanwhile, the utilization of cord blood cells is controversial and adult-derived cells may not be as successful, so numerous clinicians have begun working with stem cells that are acquired from umbilical cord blood. This review epitomizes a change in outlook from what has been completed with umbilical cord blood cell research and cord blood banking on the grounds that cord blood cells do not require much in the method of handling for cryopreservation or for transplantation in regenerative medicine.(Suman Kumar Ray et al. Recent Pat Biotechnol. 2022.- Pub Med)

DISEASES TREATED WITH CORD BLOOD STEM CELLS

Cord blood stem cells are revolutionizing the practice of medicine.
Today, there are over 80 diseases and illnesses being treated with cord blood stem cells.

Examples of diseases currently being treated with cord blood:
- Malignancies
Leukemia, Acute myeloid leukemia (AML), Lymphoma, Multiple Myeloma,
Hodgkin's disease, Retinoblastoma, Solid tumors

- Blood Disorders
Sickle cell anemia, Thalassemia, Aplastic anemia, Fanconi anemia,

Diamond-Blackfan anemia, Amegakaryocytosis Histiocytosis
- Other Diseases
Osteopetrosis, Evan syndrome, Immunodeficiencies, Severe combined immunodeficiency (SCID), Purine nucleoside phosephorylase deficiency, Reticular dysgenesis, Wiskott-Aldrish syndrome, DiGeorge syndrome, Kostmann syndrome, Omenn syndrome

- Metabolic Disorders
Adrenoleukodystrophy, Krabbe disease, Hunter syndrome, Hurler syndrome, Sanfilippo syndrome, Scheie syndrome, Sly syndrome, Lesch-Nyhan syndrome

When most people think about about stem cells treating disease they think of a stem cell transplant.
In a stem cell transplant, stem cells are first specialized into the necessary adult cell type. Then, those mature cells replace tissue that is damaged by disease or injury. This type of treatment could be used to:

* Replace neurons damaged by spinal cord injury, stroke, Alzheimer's disease, Parkinson's disease or other neurological problems;
* Produce insulin that could treat people with diabetes or cartilage to repair damage caused by arthritis; or
* Replace virtually any tissue or organ that is injured or diseased.

But stem cell-based therapies can do much more.

* Studying how stem cells develop into heart muscle cells could provide clues about how we could induce heart muscle to repair itself after a heart attack.
* The cells could be used to study disease, identify new drugs, or screen drugs for toxic side effects.

Any of these would have a significant impact on human health without transplanting a single cell.

Theoretically , there is no limit to the types of diseases that could be treated with stem cell research. Given that researchers may be able to study all cell types they have the potential to make breakthroughs in any disease.

Chapter 11

Inflammaging according to Orthomolecular Biohacking

«You cannot dry water with water, you cannot extinguish fire with fire; therefore, you cannot fight evil with evil».
Lev Tolstoy

Inflammaging is a form of chronic low-grade inflammation, not associated with infection, that develops during aging. What triggers it are mainly signals from within the body that chronically activate the immune system, for example, the presence of cell debris or oxidized proteins. This chronic activation promotes a response at the metabolic level that until middle age is essential for the survival of the body. However, it often hap-pens that during aging the inflammatory response increases to harmful levels. To this can be added the accumulation of «aged» cells, the reduction in the ability to resolve inflammation, and, according to the so-called «garbaging theory» (from garbage), the progressive reduction in the ability to eliminate cellular debris, all phenomena that increase the levels of in-flammation associated to aging.

"META INFLAMMATION"

Excess malnutrition (i.e., that type of malnutrition that depends on an excess of nutrients) can also contribute to the development of chronic inflammatory states. This specific type of chronic inflammation is associated with metabolic disorders such as obesity and type 2 diabetes and is called «metabolic inflammation» or «meta inflammation».

THE MOLECULES RELATED TO INFLAMMATION.

The most important molecules among those associated with inflammatory processes include cytokines, for example, interleukins (ILs) 2, 4, 5, 6, 9,

10,12 and 17A, GM-CSF (Granulocyte-Macrophage Colony-Stimulating Factor), TNF-α (Tumor necrosis factor α) and interferon (IFN) α and γ. Another molecule associated with inflammation is C-reactive protein (CRP). Its production is stimulated by cytokines such as IL-6, and its presence is considered a trustworthy signal of inflammation even in low-grade chronic inflammation.

Thanks to Professor Adolfo Panfili, a leader in the field of robotic, regenerative and orthomolecular biohacking medicine, a multimodal approach to regenerative medicine, based on the use of fat stem cells, isolated and expanded, for the treatment of bone matrix regeneration and prevention of cartilage degeneration (osteoarthritis), in optimal repair in clinical situations of osteoporosis is finally available and accessible.

No more inefficient fat centrifuging. In the treatment of joint degeneration, but only stem cells isolated and expanded in «clean room» from FSV (vascular stromal fraction). These are stem cells from subcutaneous fat that are the basis of the new therapy for osteoarthritis (OA).

OA is a degenerative process that affects at least 15% of the world's population and predominantly affects individuals in adulthood or young people who overstress their joints, such as professional athletes. Hip and knee osteoarthritis is considered the eleventh leading global cause of disability, as joint pain results in a disability that affects the individual's daily activities, with serious repercussions in the social and health sphere.

Data released by the WHO reveal that the 70 million people in Europe who suffer from Osteoarthritis produce an annual cost of 80 billion euros in treatment and disability management. This figure is set to double within the next 20 years, even as life expectancy increases.

Osteoarthritis is an expression of the progressive degenerative process that afflicts cartilage and thus, indirectly, joints and their function. Classic symptoms such as pain, joint stiffness, muscle tension, and instability induce the patient to immobility in an attempt to avoid pain, resulting in the production of a depressive state that worsens the overall picture.

The progression of the disease follows a development parallel to the aging of chondrocytes, cells that make up cartilage and that do not regenerate well after age 50 or following trauma damage. Treatments used to date, such as anti-inflammatory drugs (NSAIDs), intra-articular injections of fat centrifuged cells, platelet gel, and hyaluronic acid, have been minimally successful in counteracting the symptoms, but certainly not in intervening in the degenerative process of cartilage tissue.

In addition, taking drugs has led to an increase in gastrointestinal and cardiac diseases.
Osteoarthritis is therefore a degenerative problem that sees regenerative medicine, and therefore stem cells, as the only sustainable approach. Specifically, the stem cells that have the ability to differentiate into chondrocytes are mesenchymal cells, whose elective source is adipose tissue because it is easy to harvest and is always available. The ability to differentiate into chondrocytes makes stem cell therapy regenerative because, once injected near the injury, they differentiate into new cells that replace obsolete or damaged ones by renewing tissue. The breakthrough in this direction was marked by the publication of the report of the 54-month, European Union-funded ADIPOA study, with 12 European orthopedic centers united in a consortium coordinated by the University Center of Montpellier. This multicenter study, in addition to confirming the safety and efficacy of using stem cells, derived from adipose tissue and expanded, in the treatment of knee osteoarthritis, also defined the ideal dosage for a single intra-articular injection.
The study put the ideal amount of fat stem cells to be injected in a single injection at 10 million and also indicated the benefits that this dosage brings. Reduction in disability and improvement in quality of life, as measured by the WOMAC (the Western Ontario and McMaster Universities Arthritis Index) rating scale, showed a significant improvement in pain of up to 40%, with the KOOS (Knee injury and Osteoarthritis Outcome Score) scale of 30% while 50% in the VAS index.
This study indirectly affirmed that the use of fat in osteoarthritis is fruitless unless the mesenchymal stem cells in it are isolated and cultured. Indeed, it is enough to consider that if one were to obtain about 10 million cells adipose tissue stem cells without proceeding to cell culture in the laboratory, one would have to utopianly take about 2 liters of fat from the patient to perform a single treatment.

OB ADSC HAIR TRANSPLANT

A natural hair-strengthening treatment based on the use of autologous adipose tissue stem cells and transplantation in real time. With this unique approach, it is possible to combat the process of miniaturization and hair loss. HAIRSKILL is an innovative, efficaceous and safe method based on the use of adipose tissue stem cells (ADSCs) of autologous origin, that is, obtained from the fat of the individual who will undergo the treatment.

Benefits

- This is a natural method that does not involve injecting artificial components into your skin.
- It is a very accurate combined Stem Cells/ minimally invasive surgery technique: the necessary fat can be harvested on an outpatient basis.
- It is an efficaceous and safe method that is also suitable for young people who want to take action before surgery becomes the only viable route.

Directions

- The treatment is efficacious even if the bulb is irreversibly compromised. It is therefore a viable option for everyone.
- In addition, it can be an excellent solution against androgenetic alopecia and female alopecia.
- What makes this possible is the regenerative component inherent in stem cell treatment.

Results

- The first results are visible in 1 month and gradually increase over time.
- In addition, treatment with adipose tissue stem cells makes hair transplantation easier because it strengthens and prepares the scalp and stimulates grafting into the bulb.

Note: Treatment efficacy is subject to genetics, skin conditions, age and lifestyle. For these reasons, results can vary from individual to individual.

The combined regenerative technique is based on the implantation of mesenchymal stem cells obtained from one's own adipose tissue and the synergy of minimally invasive implantation. The procedure is simple and painless:

- Collection and Sampling: 20cc of fat is taken during a simple outpatient session (quick and painless).
- Extraction and Expansion: Bioscience Institute laboratories perform stem cell extraction from harvested fat. The extracted cells are expanded in about 12 days. The lab produces about 20 tubes of cells, part of which will be used for the required treatment (or several different treatments).

→

- Synergistic implant treatment: Expanded cells are injected into the tissue being treated. The injected cells release specific growth factors and promote tissue regeneration and accelerate the rooting of multiple implants.
- Cryopreservation: Remaining tubes can be frozen and cryopreserved for 3 years at the customer's request. Cryopreservation ensures use for new and future Regenerative Medicine treatments.

Chapter 12
Ozone: a planet to discover

All diseases, pain and suffering are caused by an alteration of mitochondrial functionality induced by an insufficient supply of oxygen at a cellular level.

(Arthur C Guyton - President of the American Physiology Society)

EBOO THERAPY AND ASSOCIATED THERAPIES

I have been successfully dealing with 360 degree ozone therapy for more than four decades. I have accumulated an enormous quantity from a statistical point of view of cases treated with less than exciting outcomes and I have come to the conclusion that oxygen ozone therapy represents the ideal solution for treating with success and safety a wide range of diseases. Ozone has a great oxidative capacity that can be modulated based on the most diverse therapeutic targets.

It is a molecule that behaves in a very democratic manner because it makes no distinction between castes and represents the ideal tool for defeating germs, bacteria, viruses, fungi and spores.

The never experienced administration of ozone is a successful medical practice that acts on the defense mechanisms of the immune system, deactivating the attacking pathogenic germs and strengthening the system of the large small immune defense. the operating mode of ozone therapy biologically mimics the mechanism of action of the human immune system Producing hydrogen peroxide.. Anyone knows the importance of the ozone layer which in the stratosphere protects life from harmful radiation as well as violets therefore it is easy to understand its decisive strategic effect on the life and health of the planet. It is far 1857 Werner Semen created the first equipment for the production of ozone and the first scientific report on the effects of ozone used therapeutically for blood purification dates back to 1870. EBOO therapy (extracorporeal blood oxygenation and ozonation) is a uni-que form of therapy that heals and detoxifies by stimulating oxygen metabolism, activating the immune system and

eliminating viruses, fungi, bacteria, yeasts and protozoa. The most advanced form of ozone treatment available today: a single session can actively detoxify several liters of blood using a fresh, continuous flow of ozone.
Ozone therapy is re-emerging in contemporary medicine and gaining renewed interest among patients!

EBOO (Extracorporeal Blood Oxygenation and Ozonation) therapy is a unique form of therapy that heals and detoxifies by stimulating oxygen metabolism, activating the immune system, and eliminating viruses, fungi, bacteria, yeast, and protozoa. The most advanced form of ozone treatment available today, a single session can actively detoxify several litres of blood using a fresh, continuous flow of ozone.
Ozone therapy is re-emerging in contemporary medicine and is gaining renewed interest among patients!

HOW DOES IT WORKS
Ozone increases tissue oxygenation by infusing the mitochondria with oxygen, resulting in increased energy. To the extent that ozone enhances blood flow, it relieves pain and inflammation. It also up-regulates antioxidant enzyme defenses, scavenging excess free radicals, which is key in rejuvenation and overall health.

EBOO BENEFITS
EBOO, which stands for extracorporeal blood oxygenation and ozonation is transforming the use of ozone in treating toxicity and chronic illness. For over a century, this form of ozone therapy has effectively and safely been utilized as a part of an overall treatment plan for:

* Cardiovascular disease
* Diabetes
* Lyme disease
* Chronic hepatitis
* Herpes
* Chronic fatigue syndrome
* Chemical sensitivity
* Macular degeneration
* Chronic bladder conditions
* Colitis
* Autoimmune diseases
* Crohn's disease

BEST OZONE TREATMENTS NEEDED

The number of treatment sessions and the ozone dosage administered will depend on your overall health, age, and the main condition you are suffering from. Treatments are administered once a week, and typically speaking, patients can expect to notice an improvement between the 2nd and 4th session, with full antioxidant defense mechanisms activated by the 4th treatment. Depending on your healthcare provider's recommendation, the cycle can be repeated every 3-4 months as needed.

EBOO THERAPY IS SAFE

Ozone has been proven to be extremely safe, with minor irritation to the respiratory system, if inhaled. There are no discernable side effects and the treatment is minimally invasive. That being said, if you have been diagnosed with certain conditions, please speak to a professional before proceeding with the medical use of ozone. These may include the acute and chronic tendency for bleeding/hemophilia, pregnancy, photosensitivity (or patients currently taking photo-active medicines), active diverticulitis, active diverticulosis, low platelet count, porphyria (UV blood irradiation), uncompensated hyperthyroidism (graves status), thyrotoxicosis, a known deficiency of the glucose-6-phosphate enzyme (G6PD), asthma, severe cardiovascular instability, uncompensated diabetes, acute alcohol intoxication, massive and acute hemorrhage or apoplectic stroke, thrombocytopenia less that 50,000, serious coagulation disorders, severe hypertension condition, convulsive states, hemochromatosis, ozone intolerance, ozone allergy.

Ozone Therapy Pre-Procedure Guidelines

EBOO will not impair your ability to drive, work or complete regular daily tasks, however, please follow these doctor-recommended guidelines when considering EBOO therapy:

* Hydration is important. Please increase water intake and eat beforehand.
* Notify your physician if you have experienced difficulty drawing blood in the past
* Review recommended resources to enhance your knowledge of medical ozone
* Notify your physician of drug allergies and medication changes

EBOO in my Regenerative Clinic

Extracorporeal Blood Oxygenation and Ozonation (EBOO) is transforming the use of ozone in treating toxicity and chronic illness. EBOO is the most advanced ozone therapy, and can even be more effective than multi-pass high dose ozone therapy.

EBOO uses a dialysis filter to clean blood from the debris of destroyed germs, heavy metals, fungus, etc., and to ozonate the blood in stages. Blood is drawn from one patient's vein, going through the filter, gets ozonated, and then reintroduced into the patient via another vein. The entire process happens within a closed system to eliminate the possibility of contamination in just 45 minutes!

Ozone has been used for generations and is known to have beneficial effects in killing bacteria and viruses, neutralizing toxic substances. The results of using ozone therapy, especially systemic ozone, in treating illness and infection are well documented. While several other methods of ozone therapy are available, EBOO offers the most efficient treatment in the world up to date.

Ozone Therapy works great by itself only, but you can combine it with other procedures available in our clinic for a stronger effect (e.g. PRP, Stem Cells Therapy).

Ozone Therapy is useful in a great amount of disorders:

* JOINT PAIN (Knees, Lower back, Hip, Shoulder, Elbow, Neck)
* INFLAMMATORY CONDITIONS (Arthritis, Bursitis, Nephritis, Cholecystitis, Pancreatitis, Proctitis, Cystitis)
* AUTOIMMUNE DISEASES (Fibromyalgia, Lupus, Rheumatoid Arthritis, Raynauds Disease, Scleraderma, Multiple Sclerosis, Crohn's disease, Ulcerative Colitis)
* VIRAL INFECTIONS (HIV, Hepatitis, Influenza, Herpes simplex/zoster, Mononucleosis, Measles Infections, Viral Pneumonia, Lyme Disease)
* BACTERIAL INFECTIONS (Pneumonia, Wound Infections, Septicemia (staph, strep, pneumococcus), Peritonitis, Recurrent skin infections (furunculosis), E-coli, Necrotizing infections)
* CARDIOVASCULAR DISEASES (Heart conditions, Peripheral vascular disease, Gangrene, Vascular headaches, Deep Vein, Thrombosis, Claudication, Diabetic Ulcers, Thrombophlebitis)

→

* EYE DISEASES (Retinitis Pigmentosa, Primary Glaucoma, Optic Nervy Dysfunction, Keratitis, Macular Degeneration, Iritis, Uveitis,)
* SKIN DISORDERS (Psoriasis, Non-healing wounds, Severe Acne, Recurrent skin infections, Eczema)
* RESPIRATORY DISEASES (COPD, Asthma, Emphysema, Sinusitis, Bronchitis, Tuberculosis)
* HEAVY METAL POISONING (Pb, Al, As, Hg)

Chapter 13
Antiaging DRIP IV with Stem Cells

«Panta Rei».

Heraclitus

Aging is a complex process associated with a reduction in the number of cells that enable the regeneration of organs and tissues: stem cells. The Anti-Aging IV Treatment (Intravenous Therapy), harnesses the properties of these cells to combat the decline in regenerative function that begins to manifest itself as early as middle age, with obvious signs and symptoms (such as wrinkles and joint problems). But that's not all, the passing of the years can also bring with it health-threatening issues while remaining silent and asymptomatic (such as chronic low-grade in-flammation); Anti-Aging IV therapy helps counteract even these asymp-tomatic phenomena.

This innovative approach is based on the intravenous administration (DRIP IV) of stem cells extracted from the Vascular Stromal Fraction (VSF) of the adipose tissue of the person who is a candidate for treatment (ADSC, Adipose-Derived Stem Cells) and multiplied (expanded) in the laboratory in special aseptic «clean rooms».

Basically, these are high-tech laboratories where mesenchymal stem cells, i.e., multipotent cells from which not only fat tissue cells but also many others, such as those of cartilage, bone, tendons, ligaments, muscles, blood vessels, and the nervous system, can originate. Not only that, mesenchymal stem cells produce collagen and elastin, (molecules critical to the health of organs such as the skin), but they exert anti-inflammatory action and modulate the activity of the immune system. Stem cells have the function of replenishing that Pool of amino acids essential for collagen elasticity and thus prevent the onset of wrinkles and stretch marks of skin senescence. Such amino acids are specifically lysine, proline, and glycine. As a result of stress, poor lifestyle habits, and dehydration, the body begins to sacrifice the most easily oxidized amino acids; in particular, the one that is consumed first is glycine, a structural amino acid that acts as a shock absorber of collagen molecules.

Intravenous administration (DRIP IV) of stem cells, amino acids, minerals and vitamins and especially vitamin C enable maximum enhancement of collagen tissue restructuring thus inhibiting senescence/aging processes.

BENEFITS

Compared with traditional approaches, ORTHOMOLECULAR BIOHACKING Anti-Aging DRIP IV therapy allows one to fight aging in a totally natural way by harnessing the regenerative capabilities of one's own mesenchymal stem cells. The use of autologous ADSCs nullifies the risk of adverse immune reactions, which is already low due to the low immunogenicity of these cells. In addition, the treatment does not involve surgery requiring general anesthesia. Finally, harvesting the fat from which to obtain stem cells can bring with it an additional advantage: removing unwanted fat deposits accumulated in so-called «trouble spots» (such as the hips and abdomen).

INDICATIONS

IV Anti-Aging therapy is indicated for anyone who wants to combat the problems associated with aging with the most innovative approach of those currently offered: by harnessing the natural properties of one's own stem cells. Signs and symptoms associated with the passing of the years include:

- skin aging
- Cartilage degeneration and joint problems
- subclinical inflammation
- memory problems
- reduction of forces

RESULTS: ALL-ROUND ANTI-AGING ACTION

OB Anti-Aging Drip IV Therapy has the ambitious goal of comprehensively counteracting aging. Results vary from individual to individual depending on the processes compromised by the passage of years. Improvements may be evident after only a few weeks, and tend to increase further . Only a preliminary assessment of the individual patient's situation can allow a more precise estimate of the hoped-for results. Several factors come into play, in particular:

- age
- the presence of pathologies

- lifestyle (e.g., diet and smoking) What are the expectations?
- Skin looking more youthful, fresh and toned
- increased tissue tone
- reduction of joint pain
- memory improvement
- improvement of mood
- increased energy available
- Combating inflammation and modulating immune defenses

Note: The quality of the biological product, and thus its therapeutic efficacy, is closely related to the patient's genetics, lifestyle and physical condition (obesity, smoking, alcohol and drugs will have a negative effect).

PROCEDURE

ADSC ANTI-AGING IV DRIP (the intravenous anti-aging Rosario therapy with adipose tissue-derived AD SC stem cells) is based on intravenous transfusion of autologous ADSCs, i.e., obtained from the person undergoing the treatment. The procedure is simple and painless:

Collection and Sampling

20cc of fat is harvested during a simple outpatient session (quick and painless).

Extraction and Expansion

Bioscience Institute laboratories perform stem cell extraction from the harvested fat and expands them in about 2 weeks.

Treatment

The expanded cells are transfused into the patient intravenously. Once in the circulation, they release growth factors, anti-inflammatory substances, collagen and elastin that promote organ and tissue regeneration and counteract inflammation.

Cryopreservation

Any remaining tubes can be frozen and cryopreserved for 3 years at the customer's request. Cryopreservation ensures the availability of stem cells for use in future OB Regenerative Medicine treatments.

Chapter 14
Longevity, regeneration Stem Cells and microbioma

Laudato sì, mi' Signore, per sora nostra matre terra, la quale ne sustenta et governa.

San Francesco di Assisi, Cantico delle Creature

In the first decade of the twenty-first century, genetic research had suggested that soon humanity would be able to defeat its oldest enemy, death. Neurodegenerative, cardiovascular, and oncological diseases seemed to be numbered. The complete encoding of the human genome, which occurred only in 2023, would allow us to identify and perhaps correct the causes of our organic decline. Living organisms are indeed intimately and unmistakably linked to the planet we call «Earth» and its cyclical nature. The succession of seasons is nothing but the visible image of what happens at the molecular level in every organism. In 2017, Jeffrey C. Hall, Michael Rosbash, and Michael W. Young received the Nobel Prize in Medicine for their discovery of the molecular mechanisms that control circadian rhythms. Plants, animals, and humans adapt their biological rhythm to the Earth's rotation axis. Even the universe, in its boundless vastness, responds to this ordered sequence of events that alternate without an apparent end. «Birth, growth, and death» constitute the backbone of every life cycle, from the humble protozoan to the brightest star. Many scholars and researchers have always been convinced that the principles underlying this «genetic program» were written within DNA, the molecule of heredity, the product of millions of years of evolution. This perspective had led to a backlash from some philosophers and humanists of the time, precisely because the specter of genetic determinism was beginning to loom. Man could foresee the cause and the exact moment of his death in advance, as well as his actual (limited and circumscribed) possibilities. The cinematic production of the second half of the twentieth century proposed dystopian futures in which the very essence of humanity would have been lost. Everything seemed to suggest that Francis Collins and Craig Venter, the two co-authors of the first draft of the human genome, would have marked the transition to a new era, one in which man would have been able to know and master the secret of life. As those reading this well know, this future - for better or for worse - has never materialized.

THE FAILURE OF HUMAN GENOME PROJECT

It took years to understand that the genetic code alone was not sufficient to explain the cyclical nature of life, just as genetic determinism was not the feared monster. In genes, in fact, there is not the date and because of our death, but only the draft, the blueprint, of what we could become. The secret of life was not found in our genes. Year after year, from July 2000 onwards, the scientific community continued to investigate the sequence of nucleotide bases, chromosome after chromosome. Some scholars had begun to harbor doubts about the role of DNA since it was now clear that only a small portion (less than 2%) was translated into proteins and enzymes. What then was the meaning of the remaining 98%? Was the secret of life hidden in that portion? Or was a new cipher yet to be discovered? These questions led to further and less conventional exploration of the DNA double helix. It began to be understood that large portions contained within chromosomes did not have a purely structural role but were able to regulate the expression of our genes themselves. It was the dawn of epigenetics.

LAMARCKIAN INHERITANCE

The epigenome, or epigenetics, is the set of all those chemical-physical variables found on the surface of DNA, which couldmodulate gene expression. Epigenetics allows our organism to adapt to the environment and to «remember and communicate» thismode of adaptation to subsequent generations. The idea that an activity or behavior could induce changes in DNA led many geneticists and evolutionary biologists to identify these modifications with the inheritance of acquired characteristics, proposed in the early nineteenth century by Jean-Baptiste de Lamarck in "Philosophie zoologique". The famous French naturalist, who clashed with Charles Darwin on the origin of species, believed that living beings were able to modify -within certain limits - their own biology to cope with the needs of the environment and then transmit these slight changes to their offspring. As a result of this recent reinterpretation, the terms «Lamarckism» and «Lamarckian inheritance» have reappeared in the international scientific literature. Studying epigenetics means understanding how the environment can modulate gene expression. This condition can be determined at two levels: directly, in the case of DNA methylation or histone proteins; in-directly, through the response of the endocrine system, which receives stimuli from the external environment and regulates the physiology of our body to respond promptly to different stress situations. Steroid hormones reach the cell nucleus coupled with their cytoplasmic receptor and modify the expression of individual genes. However, this activity does not involve any mechanism to «remember» that type of response, as in the case of methylation. Indeed, the most interesting aspect of methylation is related to its imprinting on the surface of DNA (a methyl group, namely a carbon atom and three hydrogen atoms), an «inheritable» modification that allows to remember how to behave (i.e., how to modulate the expression of that gene) in that life situation. The discovery of transgenerational transmission of inheritance through the language of epigenetics has opened new horizons in DNA research. It has been understood that the genetic code not only serves as a database (genes and proteins) but also that everything it is, starting from its physical, spatial, and surface conformation, carries different layers of «information.»

THE NEW FRONTIERS OF EPIGENETICS

Epigenetics today opens new and interesting perspectives for understand-ing the regulation of our genetic potential. But not only that. Through the study of DNA methylation in some portions, Steve Horvath was able to ac-curately calculate the biological age of a human being. Other interesting discoveries have been related to cancer treatment. Epigenetic changes can indeed reduce the expression of certain tumor suppressor genes (e.g., CDKN2A), a condition that can facilitate the transition from a healthy cell to a cancerous one. Just as the loss of functionality of specific genes that re-pair DNA (e.g., MGMT, BRCA1) may be due to epigenetic causes. There are also many studies applying knowledge in the field of epigenetic modifica-tions to personalize anticancer therapies. It is no coincidence, in fact, that there is increasing talk of «precision oncology.» Epigenetics is no longer just part of the scientific language but also of the literary and humanistic one. Many of the theories that have been developed over the years, even in very distant fields such as psychology, gain with epigenetics a scientific dig-nity. The transgenerational transmission of traumas could indeed be at-tributable to DNA methylation, a biological language to remember and transfer events to subsequent generations. The study of epigenetics and its heredity could have over the next twenty years the same impact that quantum physics had on classical physics.

HOLOBIONTE SUPERORGANISM OF THE CONDOMINIUM OF LIFE

The term "holobiont" was coined in 1991 by Lynn Margulis, an American evolutionary biologist and author, to describe a biological unit made up of an organism and its associated symbionts, that is, all the organisms involved in a symbiotic relationship. This concept expands the traditional notion of an individual organism to also include the organisms that live in symbiosis with it and contribute to its survival and the performance of all its biological functions.

The genetic heritage of our species can no longer be limited to the canonical 46 chromosomes, but we must extend it to the world of microorganisms (what is currently called "microbiota") that live with us in symbiosis. In fact, we must no longer consider ourselves an organism made up of our cells alone, but a real consortium, what has been identified with the term "superorganism". We are not just our cells, but we are also the cells that live with us in a mutualistic relationship (e.g. bacteria, fungi and viruses). There are nearly 39 trillion cells in our body that do not belong to our species. They are more than our own cells. The genetic heritage that we share as Homo sapiens sapiens corresponds to approximately 25 thousand genes. The microorganisms that live in symbiosis with us share over 12 million genes. This consortium of organisms, of which we are also part, has coevolved over millions of years of coexistence. All the species that populate our body have specialized to derive objective advantages from this relationship. In our intestine, for example, serotonin, the molecule of happiness, is produced. 95% of all circulating serotonin originates in the intestine, thanks to the contribution of specific microorganisms. It remains clear that the intestine, as a protected, humid and nutrient-rich place, constitutes a real ecological niche for many of these species. Two small examples to make it clear how important we are to each other.

THE INTESTINAL MICROBIOTA

The first time I described the microbiome was in 1990 in the best seller Candida the silent epidemic: you are allergic to the 21st century with New Techniques. They took me for an alien! today it's reality! The intestine is at the center of Traditional Chinese Medicine as it plays a key role in digestion, energy regulation (Qi) and mind-body balance. Its state has always been considered an indicator of the health and well-being of the organism. Eastern tradition has developed over the centuries specific treatments aimed at restoring the energy flow and functionality of this organ through acupuncture and phytotherapy. However, we must not forget that treatment in an orthomolecular approach cannot do without beneficial practices such as Tai Chi and Qi Gong. Physical exercises encourage the harmonious flow of Qi through the body's meridians and energy points, improving blood circulation, reducing stress and promoting regular bowel function.

Today, many experiences, traditions and the most recent scientific discov-eries converge in the intestine. The centrality of this organ and its inter-connection with the brain, often referred to as the enteric nervous system, has guided research towards listening to the molecular dialogue (cross-talk) that takes place in the intestinal lumen between our cells and those of microorganisms who live in symbiosis with us. A "speech" that has many codes and many languages, precisely because this dynamic interac-tion occurs continuously and between very different species. Matter and energy flow through the blood flow, lymphatic channels and nervous tissue. Here, in light of what has just been described, it is possible to understand the rea-sons that have led entire countries, organizations and research bodies from all over the world to invest considerable sums in the study of the in-testinal microbiota.

PRECISION MEDICINE

Precision Medicine was born within important scientific disciplines such as molecular biology, pharmacogenomics, and bioinformatics, which have developed since the mid-twentieth century. Precision Medicine is an avant-garde scientific discipline still evolving today; we can say that it is based on the solid foundations of knowledge belonging to traditional medicine combined with the latest scientific and technological discoveries of our time. In the document of the Regional Foundation for Biomedical Research of the Lombardy Region (FRRB), the following definition is reported: «Pre-cision Medicine is the study of the genotypic and phenotypic characteris-tics (environment, lifestyle, etc.) of each individual, which aims to integrate such information, giving unique characteristics to complex pathologies, which can thus be diagnosed and treated more efficiently, with a clear im-pact from both a medical and socio-economic point of view.» The geno-typic characteristics, present in the definition, refer to the genetic material

of our cells and to that belonging to the thousands of microbial species that have established a mutualistic relationship with us. Similarly, the dense network of molecular communication, based on epigenetics, that allows our organism to adapt to the environment and to respond quickly and efficiently to possible changes in state, must be taken into consideration. Lifestyle, food quality, pollutants, stress, are just some of the components that impact directly and indirectly on our phenotype, on what we are today. This word is indeed used to synthesize our psycho-physical status, the result of all the interactions that have led us to this «version of ourselves.» In summary, Precision Medicine places the individual at the center, not the disease or the symptom, but examines the individual in his uniqueness and as a whole: his clinical history, his individual needs, his social and family context, as well as his preferences and values. It adopts an orthomolecular approach, with modern technologies and protocols, considering not only the physical/materialistic dimension but also the emotional, mental, and spiritual aspects, correlated precisely to health.
A human-centered Medicine!

by ***Matteo Cerboneschi*** *PhD matteo@personalnext.it*

Chapter 15
FMT Microbiome Orthomolecular Biohacking born from within

"Architecturally it could be comparable to a very crowded and dangerous public condominium".

Adolfo Panfili, 2024

The microbiota represents the set of all the individual microorganisms - from bacteria, to fungi, to protozoa to viruses - that coexist with our organism without damaging it. The microorganisms that make up the microbiota are even ten times more numerous than the cells in our body. It is important to monitor the microbiota. As it represents a real shield against pathogens that could invade the skin, oral cavity, digestive tract and vagina.

Its robustness influences the state of health. In particular, the intestinal microbiota is a fundamental element for the development of the immune system and immunotolerance (the ability not to react against harmless elements). It also plays a fundamental role in the digestion and absorption of some food components (fibres and minerals), in the synthesis of some vitamins and amino acids, in the production of substances that regulate immune and metabolic responses, in the detoxification of potentially harmful substances (including carcinogens) and in the inactivation of some drugs.

In some situations, however, pathogens can take over, proliferating to the point of triggering disorders even outside the digestive system, such as urinary tract infections or bacterial vaginosis.

These and other dysbiosis (alterations of the microbiota) characterize both acute inflammation of the gastrointestinal tract and other conditions associated with inflammation, including so-called inflammaging (inflammation associated with aging).

INTESTINAL AND VAGINAL MICROBIOTA

The human microbiota lives in different body districts: in the oral cavity, stomach, small intestine and colon; in the ear; in the nose and lung; in the urinary tract; in the vagina; and also on the skin.
When we talk about intestinal microbiota we are referring in particular to the microbes that live in the intestine, a community that is approximately 10 times more abundant than the human cells of the body and whose genome (the intestinal microbiome) contains 100 times more genes than the human genome .
This community, also known as the "intestinal flora", is concentrated above all in the colon, where as many as 100 billion bacteria are found in every gram of intestinal contents.
The set of microbes that live in the vagina is called vaginal microbiota. Their genome is the vaginal microbiome.

Fecal microbiota transplantation (FMT) is now established as an effective treatment for Clostridioides difficile infection (CDI), restoring the diversity and function of the intestinal microbiome. The usefulness of FMT is currently being studied in relation to other immune-mediated diseases, such as allergic diseases, inflammatory bowel diseases and autoimmune diseases. Clinical studies in these areas are ongoing, and the altered gut microbiota (dysbiosis) often observed in these pathologies provides a rationale for the application of FMT to restore the microbiome. However, there is controversy over the benefit-risk balance as it relates to the use of FMTs in conditions other than CDI. In this Pros and Cons article we present the arguments for and against the use of FMT in immune-mediated diseases, such as allergic diseases. We further identify research gaps and recommend how these can be addressed in future studies.

FMT represents a promising paradigm for treating conditions in which the gut microbiome and dysbiosis make clear contributions to the pathophysiology However, in chronic conditions where there is uncertainty regarding the ecological factors driving dysbiosis, the timing of its development and its causal contribution to disease, the rationale for using FMT may be weak and the risk-benefit ratio unfavorable.

Chapter 16

OB Program to get back in shape and lose weight without drugs

«Life is a molecular interaction.»
Linus Pauling

Being fit and healthy also means living without subjugation to medication. Wellness is the quintessence of self-respect and essential rules that start with the style of life. Proper nutrition, the right amount of physical activity and rest are necessary tools for better living. Medications save lives, especially in emergencies, but should be avoided when unnecessary and in any case consumed very sparingly and in moderation. Finally, a distinction should be made between chemical-pharmacological molecules and supplements (amino acids, vitamins, minerals, herbal products, etc.).

One in three intoxications is caused by medicines. Medications are used to treat, but they are also the main contributors to poisonings worldwide. In fact, drugs are the subject of 34 percent of the 67,000 requests for advice received by poison control centers each year. And children are particularly at risk: among all types of intoxication, not only drug-related, 44 percent of cases concern children under 5 years old, according to data also published in the National Epidemiological Bulletin of the Italian National Institute of Health, but as we know, the world is one large country, and Italy is only an tip of the iceberg.

Medications are formidable tools for our health, but they should be used with care because they can have side effects that are sometimes serious. Prevention to be implemented through enhanced operator training and pharmacovigilance, which should also take into account patients' age and anthropometric characteristics (weight, height, BMI, etc.). Today's reporting of adverse effects, unfortunately, is generic, and does not include data collection by age group; instead, special attention to children and the elderly is desirable. Still on the subject of drug vigilance, it is interesting to evaluate the study on notifications of suspected adverse effects of, for example, COVID-19 vaccine serums in Switzerland. In the update 16,855 suspected case notifications were analyzed. The notifications would confirm the risk-benefit profile of the vaccines. Up to Feb. 22, 2023, 10,365 suspected adverse drug reactions of 61.5 percent reported as non-serious were examined, while 6,490 suspected cases of 38.5 percent were notified to Swissmedic as serious.

In most cases, a notification contains more than one section in total and 52,404 reactions were observed and reported, which corresponds to an average of 3.11 % reactions per report. This figure must, of course, take into account the fact that under some policies of previous governments: For example, in Italy it was particularly complex to file reports on possible side effects from serum vaccination, and this was regardless of the goodness or otherwise of the prophylaxis, but in essence because the Italian state would have been caught unprepared by the Covid epidemic without appropriate emergency management health planning.

In this regard, the commendable initiative of the SIF (Italian Society of Pharmacology), which has set up a website (www.sifweb.org), on which a system for reporting adverse effects is already active, is worth mentioning. In one year more than one million reports have been collected, and these data have all been made available to institutions.

Under indictment, as far as medicines are concerned, mostly analgesics and anti-inflammatory drugs (13 percent) but also sedatives, hypnotics, antipsychotics and antidepressants (10 percent), antihistamines (8 percent), hormones (7 percent), antibiotics (6 percent), dental caries prophylaxis products (fluoride) (3 percent), antiseptics (3 percent) and even disinfectants, classified as parapharmaceuticals, associated with 6 percent of accidental intoxication cases.

Most people who resort to hospitalization because they are suffering from side effects of drugs, such as: sudden bleeding, bleeding, dermatitis, redness or other skin damage, hypotension or hypoglycemia, etc., are not able to be hospitalized.

Countless hospitalizations related to medication use or abuse. The line between drug use and abuse is often thin, subjective, and variable in that even wise and sparing use of a chemical molecule cannot avoid unexpected reactions.

Increasingly, drugs are gradually turning from «health tools» into consumer goods; take for example the blue pill of happiness, the much-lauded Sildenafil (Viagra). A simple look at numbers and statistics shows that far more euros are spent annually on hedonistic drugs than on essential illnesses.

Pharmacological Philosopher's Stone of Wellness? Through newspapers, magazines and TV, unfounded and disappointing expectations of recovery are often created among sufferers and family members. So why not try to explore the possibility of trying to get better and get back in shape without drugs?

Chapter 17

If you want to change the body, change the mind!

«Imagination is more important than knowledge and governs the world.»
Albert Einstein

Stude's statistics state that about 70 percent of the learning that takes place in the first six years of life will create the ability to acquire new information. This stage of life is also the most fertile since the point of view of imagination.

A good imagination would therefore be indispensable for early and good learning. We should devote more time and respect to creative imagination in school teachings, stimulating and developing it as much as possible until adulthood.

How many times will you have heard a parent say, «I'm worried because my child shows an incredible imagination!» or, «That child is always with his head in the clouds...,» while others seem to believe that the value of a child's imagination coincides exclusively with the ability to entertain and amuse adults. A good imagination is as valuable as a good memory and is the key to any solid culture and the strategy for solving most existential dilemmas. Characters such as Einstein and Edison were endowed with splendid imaginations. Albert Einstein in particular arrived at his scientific conclusions about space-time by mentally projecting himself into a virtual extraplanetary world, in which he was free to frolic far and wide astride pale moonbeams. His childlike regression skills helped him become a giant among intellectuals of all time.

Aging is not the worst of evils, while rather the loss of the power to visualize is.

Some people show faster recovery after serious illness and surgery following the simple administration of a placebo (from Latin = to give relief), that is, of an inert substance, completely devoid of pharmacological properties, also known as 'sugar pill' but nevertheless capable, in certain individuals with a more fervent visualization capacity, of psychologically supporting and accelerating healing. It is not uncommon that sometimes the opposite effect, termed nocebo, occurs with the use of the same substance. In this case patients present with the onset of rather serious and unpleasant side effects. In both cases it is the expectation related to the particular molecule used that makes the classic difference and justifies the ambivalence of the result.

Among the placebo-nocebo effect substances, the following should definitely be included: words, diagnoses made or not made, and the attitude of the doctor or surgeon or any other authority figure toward the patient. Peremptorily communicating to a sick person, «You only have six months to live because you have cancer,» represents unnecessary sabotage to his immune and defensive strategies, as well as being cynical and inhumane behavior.

Why not tell them that in addition to deaths caused by this disease, there are cases of people who manage to fight to conquer, perhaps painstakingly, their recovery and that their behavior deserves to be studied and imitated?

More than four thousand cases of established cures have been analyzed by the San Francisco Institute of Noetic Sciences (Sausalito) in California as part of the Neoplastic Remissions Project. This information is accessible through the Internet for anyone and especially for those who express skepticism to the possibility of cure from cancers.

According to Siegel, at least 90 percent of people who recover from a malignancy would have experienced a significant change in their quality of life prior to the recovery itself.

Accepting that an emotional event can trigger the onset of cancer is as dangerous as Columbus's belief that the Earth was round when everyone thought it was flat, which is why many prefer to talk about an initial diagnostic error, when an «unexpected» healing changes the game, rather than having to admit the possible link between mind, body and soul.

Hamer, author of the eponymous «Outbreak Theory,» had to defend his thesis before his home medical board by presenting dozens of cases of patients cured of the «Evil of the Century» without drugs, but simply by resolving the emotional conflict underlying it.

This statement is not intended to trivialize or diminish the significance of such an intense and dramatic issue, but rather to try to understand the strategies behind it.

Older people often report that they no longer have a good memory. Many of them have let their imaginations deteriorate to such an extent that their minds can no longer create images capable of adhering to the firmament of their thoughts.

Health and the mystery of healing have always fascinated mankind, which since the dawn of time has regarded it as the effect of invisible and intangible forces, to be propitiated in the presence of touchy and wrathful deities.

For a very long period of humanity, diseases and epidemics were considered expressions of divine wrath.

The healer was alone in the presence of these frightening and occult energies, he had to descend into the underworld of the psyche to access the coded language of the soul, in an internal journey, where the will of the individual had little meaning, except to pity the merciful will of a supreme and unique God to be pacified segregated in the individual viscera of the true self. **Every man can heal, and at least once in his life, unfortunately... he dies, even without the intervention of the drug, implying that this complement should not be considered an irreplaceable deterrent in the evolution of human civilization.**

Leonardo painted the Mona Lisa even without ever having taken an aspirin tablet for the headache that plagued him in his inspirational dives. Michelangelo sculpted the Pieta and decorated the entire Sistine Chapel even without ever having ingested an analgesic capsule in order to overcome the bouts of cervicobrachialgia from which he suffered (neck pain extending to the upper limbs).

Julius Caesar suffering from epilepsy certainly did not die because he had not taken diphenylhydantoin, while Jesus and his trusted disciples were fearlessly and uncontaminatedly scampering around Palestine without having undergone any vaccination...

MIRROR NEURONS

There is a so-called dark side to the power of interpersonal relationships. Specifically I am referring to mirror neurons that represent a sort of fundamental ingredient of everyone's life from a social and relational point of view.

A team at Stanford University in the United States, based on work done by Professor Rizzolatti (Director of the Parma Center for Neurophysiology and a close friend of mine) have identified mirror neurons in the anger center of the brains of male rats. Such neurons light up like neon lamps when a rodent gets into a fight, which occurs when a male is placed in another male's cage, thus violating his territory, but also occurs when he observes a fight by others.

When artificially deactivated the neurons by researchers, the rats instead become tame and are able to forget even the presence of any females.

The parallel on stereotypical human behavior is all too obvious, but let's proceed in order: given the immense popularity of violent video games or fighting contests it seems clear how aggression, even that observed as mere spectators in movie theaters, can be appeased. This is what researchers led by Mira Hao Sha write in the article published in Cells, the authoritative journal on the subject.

Even observing someone else's scuffle improves fighting technique and enables one to become more aggressive.

When aggression becomes contagious then things get complicated. Mirror neurons are involved in aggression, they have in fact been observed in a particular region of the hypothalamus, known as the anger center (Cajal's nucleus) demonstrating that we are not dealing with higher functions, but with deep and ancient cores of the phylogenetic survival of the species, structured for defense and fight.

The other two pillars are sex and food, and at this point we have to ask a question whether they too can be controlled.

Chapter 18

No pain no gain-accepting and transcending fear by overcoming it

---

«One day fear knocked at the door.
Courage went to open it and found no one.»
Martin Luther King Jr.

Did you know that there is a switch to defuse fear? It is called the EPIPHYSIS, an endocrine gland (also called the body or pineal gland) located in the interior of the skull between the eminences anterior quadrigeminal artery and joined to the encephalon by a peduncle.

It is a real crystal computer that filters frequencies and is also capable of influencing the level of leptin, GH and other hormones; in fact, it regulates the human body's daily (circadian) rhythms and helps modulate seasonal ones.

The ancients knew that the pineal gland (the epiphysis) represents a portal connecting physical reality to higher dimensions. It could be called «a bio-star portal,» a bridge between the physical and the nonphysical, between duality and immensity, between the three-dimensional brain and the Infinite Mind.

The epiphysis is an intermediary of advanced consciousness. It works in synergy with the pituitary gland to create a bridge between dimensions.

The problem for most people lies in blind acceptance of mental and three-dimensional programming. You can think positively, reflect on changes for the better, but if, deep in your mind, you doubt that this can happen, nothing will happen. Rest assured of that!

Every emotion you feel, every moment of joy or fear creates chemical ferments in the body.

Some of these messengers become stepping stones, others become obstacles. And each of them reaches the epiphysis. The epiphysis is a calcite crystal. A finely tuned, piezoelectric, similar to quartz crystal. It is a kind of filter, is a guardian on the path that connects with the Divine. It prevents the manifestation of some thoughts with negative vibrations, such as fear, doubt, anxiety, and others that do not have positive vibrations. Therefore, an intent toward which you harbor doubts cannot be included in the programming.

Doubt creates a biochemical reaction in the brain that activates a direct neural influx from the pituitary to the epiphysis and blocks the opening of the «portal» through the epiphysis.

Doubt and fear are two inhibiting frequencies that sabotage the realization of our desires.

In fact, all negative emotions are based on fear. Overcoming fear and replacing it with Love, especially self-love, deep acceptance, is what is needed to overcome duality. The epiphysis is the threshold of the Biohacker's journey descending into the unknown of the deep self by overcoming fateful trials. Remember the labors of Hercules? They are overcome with «COURAGE» that transcends «FEAR.»

The epiphysis is a system for entering the Divine; it is a complex crystalline computer that filters frequencies to conquer the alchemical elixir of awareness. NO PAIN NO GAIN. In conclusion, if you don't accept to face fear the game is not won and like in the game of the goose you start over again, until we would have karmically understood this lesson.

When aggression becomes contagious then things get complicated. Mirror neurons are involved in aggression, they have in fact been observed in a particular region of the hypothalamus, known as the anger center (Cajal's nucleus) demonstrating that we are not dealing with higher functions, but with deep and ancient cores of the phylogenetic survival of the species, structured for defense and fight.

The other two pillars are sex and food, and at this point we have to ask a question whether they too can be controlled.

Chapter 19
Laughter therapy: to change perspective point and detoxifying negative thoughts

«Always laugh when you can. It's free medicine.»
Lord Byron

Laughter is an operative mode for evading stress from a neurovegetative point of view.

ETHICS OF LAUGHTER

With humor we experience a sudden change in ns cognitive patterns (schemas) by taking advantage of the lightning-fast operational speed of lateral thinking. In other words, if we were to proceed with monochromatic and linear crystallized structured thinking, the time required to change our usual mental patterns would be exceedingly long and complex to pursue and still disturbing.
Some artists of the laughter technique (such as Greg, Lillo, Alivernini, Ferrario, etc.) innately possess these lateral semantic-expressive codes and perform at a very high level, creating a real system of public speaking that many professionals should take as a paradigm and start using it to improve inter-human empathic communication.
Laughter like a time bomb must be triggered at the right moment in the dynamics of communication, and once it explodes its deterrent is practically immense.
I have seen heads of state, leaders of multinational corporations, famous actors, and stiff, structured personalities melt away in an instant after a good laugh strategically dropped on the most appropriate target.

Definitely «Laugh Bombing» is the only form of bombing that is not only «acceptable» but necessary.
However, we must never forget that next to every great «Laugh Bomber Therapist» like Greg there is always a great co-pilot to aim and hit the target. Yes, I'm talking about Nicoletta and who else?
A stupid thing said by a smart man makes us doubt him, while a smart thing uttered by a stupid man... makes us doubt ourselves. In life almost always when we have to learn a new lesson we are forced to go through Pavlovian conditioning, that is, related to the element of suffering.
Just as puppies are taught not to pee on the carpets at home by spanking them with newspaper, it is fair to say that for us poor humans, too, «without pain there is no growth!».
It is no coincidence that Mother Nature, who is never wrong (not even when she seems to be wrong to us) has provided us with pain nerve endings in markedly greater numbers than those deputed to distill pleasure, in the ratio of 3:1.
Which would be the equivalent of saying that if you get a hammer in the head your HIFI system of perception receives it 3 times better than if. Jodie Comer decided to spend a night on fire with you after 5 tablets of Viagra!

Note: Instead, may the kind ladies have the courtesy to exchange Jodie Comer for Henry Cavill. Di Caprio, Brad Pitt, etc.

«No pain, no gain» - a heraldic motto that often towers in bodybuilding gyms where biceps are forged through toil and sweat!
Sport certainly poses to those who can grasp a variety of analogies with amatory activity, among which physical endurance is a proverbial symbol, but a copulative act is one thing, and running a marathon is another. Certainly both feats can literally lay the performer down on a candid bed at the end of the performance, but the dynamics of execution present no few obvious differences.
Try out of curiosity if you are used to practicing meditation or if you decide to start using it for better living, to precede the session by a series of full and total laughter, trying to imitate the Lone Surfer, and you will realize how much quicker and more effective access to these states of inner expansion can be and how much easier it is to maintain them.
Not surprisingly, in Tibet we refer to vigilant meditation as that moment when a fly's wing manages to glide over the edge of a sharp razor.
That somewhat nutty patient had taught me more than any textbook about

the occult significance of the thaumaturgy of laughter as a neurovegetative tonic. Laughter, especially in critical and desperate situations, liberates a whole series of endorphin mediators and neurotransmitters that can emotionally turn the most dramatic of situations upside down, all you need is the constancy to keep laughing out loud for at least ten minutes and that's it, the whole rest of your person will resonate with the initial laughter chasing away the demon of despair from your terrified and distraught minds.

Laughing makes not only the face laugh, but also the diaphragm, the viscera, improves blood circulation, and boosts immunity and greatly alkalizes cells and tissues.

To laugh, more than 60 muscles are used - for, mimic, cervical, etc., while to cry only about 20 - so isn't the real jog for the soul laughter, dear readers?

LAUGHING DOES NOT DIFFER THAT MUCH FROM MEDITATING AND PRAYING

«We do not laugh because we are happy, but we are happy because we laugh.»
A.P.

If we search PubMed, the leading search engine for biology and medicine publications, for the term meditation, nearly 10,000 titles come up:

1,000 per year in recent years, 10 years ago it was 400, 20 years ago 50 per year, 30 years ago about 30. Scientific research is realizing that our mind influences the functioning of our body and our health. Meditation reduces anxiety, depression, conflict, and aggression; reduces stress and plasma cortisol levels; normalizes metabolic syndrome (hypertension, dyslipidemia, hyperglycemia); increases telomere length (the DNA at the ends of chromosomes that shortens with each cell division, a major marker of longevity); and reduces inflammation, specifically silencing genes that promote the synthesis of NFkB, the major transcription factor that promotes the synthesis of inflammatory cytokines. A dozen studies have found that meditation reduces the inflammatory state. Meditation reduces chronic pain. A review of 20 clinical trials shows that in addition to reducing NFkB and C-reactive protein (a marker of inflammation), meditation improves a number of parameters that indicate better immune defenses.

So if prayer is hostile to you, at least laugh at it!

Fear, on the other hand, causes the release of adrenaline and norepinephrine, stress hormones that both in the water and outside of this element would diffuse with extreme rapidity, so much so that they would be sensed by opposing finfish in the span of a few seconds.

As you navigate the great sea of life it can be very helpful to know how to laugh. I often ask some of my patients to re-educate themselves to global laughter and I prescribe therapeutic laughter at least six times a day and the results believe me are fantastic, and believing is trying!

Dusty old paintings in the attic often rise to new life when they are taken to the framer to have them reframed. Similar process is achievable with any negative experience, and it is almost always possible to extrapolate its positive and amusing side. It's just a matter of direction!

In NLP (Neuro Linguistic Programming) this process is called Reframing. Transform any event into a new chance and opportunity by demonstrating resilience, willingness and adaptability to constant changes in the sur-rounding environment, continuously exploring new hypotheses in social, cultural, affective contexts.

The best therapists are those who continually learn from the school of life and are able to set the jewels of their life experiences in new and beautiful frames and pass them on to others. The concept of a therapist expands and healing is possible for anyone if communication between human beings is restored.

You are all cells of the same tissue, and for the health of each organ and the body itself, it is good that the dialogue between the parts is never interrupted. Never before has silence become synonymous with stillness and lifelessness. Laughing well reunites the fragments and enables one to gain orthomolecularity, synonymous with wholeness.

In Panfhealing seminars, the exercise of therapeutic laughter is one of the cornerstones on which the individual metamorphosis induced by Reframing hinges, and in the group it is always very successful; after practicing it, people seem to regain the joy of living so much so that at the end of the seminar they look like different people and by looking at her face their faces appear more serene, relaxed and full of confidence.

Laughing is easier than you may assume, simply try to imitate someone else who is already laughing and you are done. If you hear someone laugh-ing and his laughter pleases you, approach him without reservation by openly declaring that you would like to clone and learn his beautiful laugh-ter. Identify and memorize well the physiology of the state of mind related to laughter and make use of it to recreate it when there is neither need; in fact, only by modifying the physiology of your negative emotional states will you be able to improve the level of performance and.... most importantly you will not be devoured by the sharks you may encounter along your route!

HE WHO LAUGHS THE MOST LIVES THE LONGEST

«You have to laugh before you can be happy,
Not to risk dying without having laughed.»
Jean de La Bruyère

Quarter past four!
Norman had arrived transfixed as usual to yet another appointment, late for a change!
His life had always been all about rushing from one thing to the next, but this was the one time where he could surely indulge in a Latino delay, to put a Mexican to shame-no one was going to scold him!
Since 3pm at the testing laboratory, in an anonymous yellow envelope was waiting the verdict regarding the future of his life.
The eschatological and glacial diagnosis of the anatomo-pathologist was all too clear and sharp: «Ewing's Sarcoma» with scattered metastases!
Oh yes! for once he had really done well to take it easy; his head in the noose of the impending news. After all, he was not in such a hurry to put it there. After all, he thought, «what the eye doesn't see, heart doesn't grieve!». So it happened that the fateful spring snapped, and Norman decided to cure himself by devoting himself to laughter, beginning to attend comedy shows intensively: cabarets, hilarious films, jokes, trying to rediscover the funny side of life, which he had forgotten for so long and which perhaps, according to Dr. Hamer's theories, had cost him that nice little gift of bone cancer.
In that moment of mental satire, he caught himself wondering why, and since when, he had chosen to go with the anxiety and anguish instead of the harmony of gay lightheartedness that seemed to distinguish him in the first phase of his life. Now in his 50s, he no longer recognized himself in that sad and sullen stranger. He was the specter of what he never thought he would become... how strange he could no longer even remember when and because he had given himself the ultimate global heart and bladder laugh, the kind that can make you vibrate from head to toe, to the point

where you lose control of your sphincters... in short, to pee yourself to be more realistic and explicit... could that ever be possible?
Was he getting sad, or had life suddenly become a dark tunnel from which to exit as soon as possible aboard a tumor, rather than by subway?
That terrible diagnosis still rumbled in his eardrums like a blacksmith's mallet forging glowing iron.
Those succinct, lapidary words written in that cryptic language that only doctors know how to use so well when it is needed to frighten the condemned to death... progressively terrified him, taking away his will to breathe. Why to him of all people that ominous message, sharper than a razor, which just by uttering it already foreshadowed the roll of the cancer surgeon's scalpel sliding over the Langhans lines of his fear-tightened skin?

Chapter 20
The Journey of the Biohacker

«The first degree of heroism is to overcome fear and self-mastery.»
Gian Piero Bona (Walk with the Devil, 1983)

Human beings have been telling stories since the dawn. We tell stories to teach lessons, to share messages, to set examples. Stories are the means by which we organize and communicate the meaning of events and experiences; they are the bridge, the link between culture and the individual.

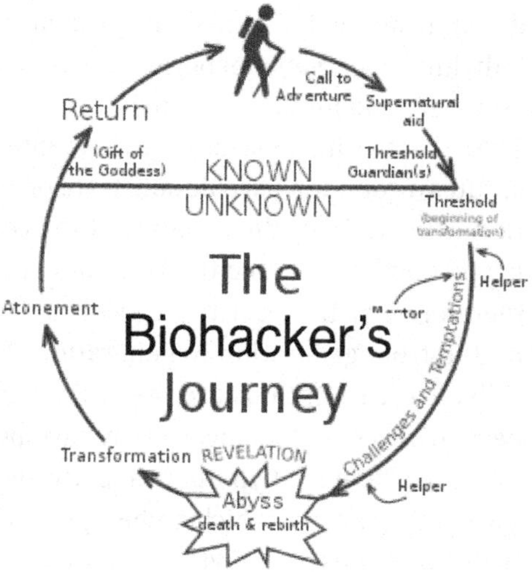

Stories are also central to the development of the concept of self-image and of identity; according to some authors, identity is precisely a form of narrative, allowing us to interact and react to the world, to life events, and to possess a unified identity that remains constant despite the passage of time and the succession of multiple life events.

There are stories that speak of loss, the end of love, bereavement, but they also speak of joy, of loves and dreams coming true and the ability to survive despite pain, the ability to adapt, change and be happy despite difficulties. Storytelling, the telling of one's own story (which is about events experienced in the first person but also about events that affect people close to us), is a fundamental component of diagnosis and therapeutic intervention, and every therapist makes use of it. The stories we hear also can play

an important role in the construction of our identity and the way we view the world and life.
The stories we hear, read, and see on a screen allow us to identify ourselves, to mirror ourselves, to recognize ourselves in one of the characters or events narrated, and it is this mirroring function of stories that is the secret of their fascination.
Most stories we read in a book or see in a movie reflect a particular structure, that from the «hero's journey» as conceptualized by Joseph Campbell.
Joseph Campbell, a historian of religions and comparative mythology, as well as' a profound connoisseur of Jung's theories, develops his reflections in search of connections between mythology and analytical psychology.
To better understand Campbell's proposed structure, we must have in mind some basic elements of Jungian thought.
According to Jung, the collective unconscious is a part of the psyche that differs from the individual unconscious in that it is not derived from the individual's personal experiences, but whose contents are the same everywhere and for all individuals.
The collective unconscious is thus identical for all human beings and constitutes a common psychic substrate of a suprapersonal nature.
According to Jung, the contents of the collective unconscious have never been conscious, unlike the contents of the individual unconscious, and therefore owe their existence solely to the fact that they have been transmitted from generation to generation. The elements that constitute the collective unconscious are the archetypes. Archetypes are common (indeed «collective») «images» that have been present since ancient times; they are a kind of «hypothetical patterns.»
Two of the ways in which archetypes are expressed (and thus made partially conscious) are myth and fable. Campbell sees all myths, fables or folktales, as variations of a single grand story-the monomyth-in that there is a common pattern underneath the narrative elements that goes beyond their geographical origin or the time of their creation. The pattern identified by Campbell is expressed particularly well by the journey that heroes, the protagonists of myths, stories and films, face.

THE CALL TO ENTERPRISE

The Biohacker's journey begins with the «call to adventure,» presented to the Biohacker by the messenger; if the Biohacker decides to undertake the path will find himself having to leave the world that is known to him, familiar to him, and having to venture into a space that is unknown to him.

MEETING WITH TH E W ISE MAN

The Biohacker's journey continues with an encounter with the «mentor or wise old man.».Between Biohacker and mentor an alliance is created that will allow the Biohacker to progress and complete his journey. On the Biohacker's path there are then a series of difficulties, trials and changes, (which Campbell referred to as first second and third thresholds) but also encounters with characters who offer help.

THE ABYSS, REVELATION AND THE ALCHEMICAL E LIXIR

The Biohacker will then encounter on the way the most complex moment of his journey, the moment of the abyss. The moment which will then also turn out to be the moment of the revelation of the rediscovered alchemical elixir, of the discovery of something new in the story and especially in the character of the Biohacker; this is the moment of the «death and rebirth» dynamic.

THE RETURN TO THE O RIGINS

At this point, the Biohacker is transformed by the journey he has taken and the time comes for him to reconcile with the world that was unknown to him before his departure, to reconnect with his past now that he has gained a new perspective and new abilities; it is the time of «coming home.»

Thus in myths, fairy tales, folk legends and today, in movies-all representations of the collective psyche-we find the pattern of individual destinies that each of us will embody in a story.

Chapter 21
Emotional OB

With Orthomolecular Biohacking it is possible to manipulate your emotions and moods in an instant, just as you change your clothes, just as you can discover your best teacher in your worst enemy!
Thank him, what are you waiting for?

(Adolfo Panfili)

Like an old wounded elephant that does not forget, the individual subconscious "ties its finger" on even the slightest abuse suffered during pre- and post-natal existence. Emotional conflicts for humans are cumulative, and just like BOTs they are capable of producing interests. The investment of psychic energy or the drive towards any object: fantasies, desires, people, objectives, ideas, social groups or even towards one's own self is defined as Catexis, (from the Greek: catexo, "I occupy")
Each new emerging conflict will therefore be automatically compared with previous emotional experiences, adding to these in an exponential and progressive manner, like a snowflake which, sliding down the slope of life, becomes a real avalanche capable of overwhelming everything that stands in his way.
Having suffered an affront, violence, physical or verbal aggression, exerts a notable influence on the level of the individual subconscious memory determined by negative thoughts which can resurface in the most unexpected moments, triggering a defensive physiology, acting as an alarm stimulus. for the sensory system.
The subconscious does not reason, but simply reacts to feelings by creating cathexis, or sequential actions and responses, characterized by the release of psychic energy related to complexes of ideas closely associated with emotions and other physical factors, so that when an idea is recalled to mind, it is automatically associated with the painful or rewarding experience already experienced, reactivating and updating its metabolic aspects.
The Central Nervous System (CNS), through the Reticular Activator System (SRA), carries out an emotional filter action and retains as unmistakable

signs any information coming from the external world, including previous emotions, to then release them again in the most critical moments below. form of anxiety, irritability, depression, resentment, or as positive uplifting and constructive feelings.

In a unit of time you are literally bombarded by a myriad of stimuli and the brain can only focus on a narrow range of this data.

Through this network, from which the term reticular comes, only those data deemed interesting for the brain pass like fish in the ocean of objective reality, which therefore develops its own extremely subjective and in any case partial observation point of the universe, deciding to whom and what to listen to. Think of two football teams competing in a stadium, clearly the players of one team will be positively stimulated by the encouragement of their fans, while they will be much less attentive and sensitive to those of their opponents. In this situation it is precisely the RSA (reticular activator system) that allows this listening selectivity. With the name E.P. (Bridging Emotions) is intended to connote those emotions and feelings of such subjective, and not absolute, conflictual meaning as to be able to influence the behavior of the individual, both in the mind and in the body to such an extent as to create a sort of bridge between the psyche and the soma (body). Even opposing feelings such as love, esteem, gratitude, trust, can create positive anchors and act as a springboard to achieve joy and fulfillment. Successful and healthy people are able to make the most of this sort of self-programming, developing the winning ability to never consider their emotions and symptoms wrong, rather considering them as precious signals. Opposing a negative or positive emotion is equi-valent to trying to stop an avalanche with a teaspoon! Instead, it is wiser to cultivate esteem and appreciation for what the body intends to commu-nicate through sensory channels.

Like a buoy in a sailing regatta, these emotions are pivots around which the subject's existence often revolves and develops. For example, having had an emotional disappointment or a betrayal by your partner can lead you to choose as your next partner a person with characteristics diame-trically opposed to the previous one. It is equally possible, after having been loved in a family where one grew up in the spirit of trust, communi-cation and collaboration, to find a partner who perfectly resonates with this form of life, and acquire more chances of being happy.

This alliterative mechanism does not correspond to the true expectations of those who have suffered the wrong, but corresponds to a sort of defensive retaliation. Choosing a gentle and calm companion will be an excessive alliterative reaction and will certainly not reflect the real vocation of a cou-

ple for those who have been burned by suffering.
For purely defensive purposes, the exact opposite of the situation that caused the conflict to arise is often chosen.
This conduct can be a source of great unhappiness, which is why in the Orthomolecular Biohacking approach we work by trying to bring past conflicts, emotions and feelings to the surface to let them melt like snow in the sun, reducing them through the acquisition of a new awareness. Repressed emotions are often the cause of major diseases. Impressions made on the subconscious are able to influence your world, including your health.

THE EMOTIONS THAT MAKE US SICK ARE THE SAME THOSE THAT CAN SAVE US

Man needs laughter as an outlet, animals do not, because they are generally subjected to less mental stress, not being inclined to become embittered or worn out by a certain situation;
In fact, they do not feel guilty or burdened by psychological responsibilities.

(Adolfo Panfili - Course for training managers in Orthomolecular Biohacking)

The feelings, emotions and words that negatively influence the individual should absolutely not be ignored, and the messages they try to convey must be listened to and analysed.
Often the intensity of the pain that accompanies them makes those who experience them incapable of interpreting the esoteric message that lies behind them, missing a further opportunity for personal and karmic development. Use these sad sisters as precious compasses on a dark and foggy night and they will be able to show you the safest route, but do not challenge them by underestimating them, because they would know how to undermine your future. Sign an armistice treaty with these gentle ladies and they will become your teachers and you the faithful disciples who will be able to distill from the must the most delicate wine of happiness...
As? Finding the silver lining in the darkest of the following situations:

-HATE
-FEAR
-CRITICISM
-ANGER

-RESENTMENT
-ENVY
-FRUSTRATION
-GUILT
-SOLITUDE (imposed)
-ANXIETY
-DOUBT
-JEALOUSY
-SELFISHNESS
-TYRANNY

Chapter 22
We are made of the same stuff as our dreams

"Our souls travel spaces of Life
not commensurable by the hourglass of time
invented by man to fence the sand of the ocean of the universe"

(Adolfo Panfili)

One cannot help but agree with this statement by Shakespeare, in fact the human body is not a Sicilian cannoli stuffed with organs, nor even the random assembly of replaceable biochemical molecules.
A body is not a simple agglomeration of receptors, cells and organs, but much more.
A sort of intelligent memory updates and makes us aware of any event that is occurring or has already occurred, or is about to occur in the entire human organism.
Many have tried, without success, to track down the director of this exciting and endless show that the adventure of life has been offering us for millions of years. In the last century, even a group of enthusiastic scientists even dedicated themselves to "weighing" people, a few moments before and a few moments after their death, to check for any lightening related to an escape of the soul. However, the experiment at least provided the information that if man has a soul, it probably weighs nothing.

Simply think that in a single respiratory act you inhale and exhale 10 to 22 atoms that originate in every cell of your organism from the heart, to the kidney, to the brain tissue, etc. By carrying out appropriate studies with radioactive marking isotopes you would realize that in a certain sense everyone also shares their organs with their neighbor, in an atomic sense.

At this very moment in each of you the alchemy of the species ensures that there reside at least a million of the atoms that were once housed in the body of Christ, or Napoleon, Buffalo Bill, Putin or Trump or any other person that you have decided to think about.

In the space of one calendar year, over 98% of the atoms in your body that you are using will be completely replaced.

At an atomic level, in less than five days the gastric mucosa is completely renewed, while in a month the skin that covers your body is completely regenerated.

How much more do you want to suffer? Decide it for yourself and decide it now without blaming others, if you still avoid this existential crossroads.
Every change in awareness or quantum leap requires the supply of external energy to your system, it means dying to metaphorically be reborn in another dimension.
Do you have an unsatisfactory relationship behind you, but are you afraid of ending it because the simple idea of living alone scares you?
If you are tired of your profession, look for another job that enjoys you and makes you happy!
If your energy is low and you feel tired, fatigued and stressed, it's time to tap into a higher level of health and well-being.
To quench your cosmic thirst for life, it is up to you only to choose whether to use a thimble, a glass or a tanker...

Chapter 23

Let's use Empowerment to deal with change

«You have power over your own mind.
If you want to change external events, change yourself. Realize this and you will find strength.»

Simona Scarpati (simona.scarpati@mac.com)

«Empowerment,» an untranslatable term in Italian, has its deepest roots in Socratic maieutics. One will be able to find answers that are generated directly by ourselves, birthing them and Making them finally come out, because every answer is already in us. To cope in the best way, using tools that are within us, with the exceptionality' of the historical period in which we find ourselves, is configured as a path that is as necessary as ever, especially for all those who need to find new resources and energy that springs from our inexhaustible resources, which only need to be slated.
Learning to use empowerment for change through a path of biohacking offers the possibility of overcoming obstacles, taboos and discomforts only by becoming aware of our personal power, reactivating the Biohacker within each of us. It is a path that will make it possible to deal with discomfort by transforming it into opportunity, to benefit from what until yesterday was a burden and/or discomfort. For years the analysis and verification of phenomena related to the expression of worries, thoughts, doubts, fears and in general to the production and manifestation of all sorts of emotional ballast has been going on unabated. Anxiety and a sense of inadequacy prevent people with enormous creative potential from believing in themselves. Education, social roles, and obligations to those who generated us do the rest, and we often live a life that is not our own, playing a character that we do not identifies or represents. Unhappiness turns brilliant minds into sad golems, but through awareness each of us will be able

to transform, as in an alchemical process, any inner dross into valuable visionary energy. A true virtuous process will be set in motion, for there is nothing more exciting than discovering a light and sharing it with others. A great improvement in self-esteem can be achieved by getting in touch with a deeply wise and resilient part of us.
Below are the goals that are achieved:

- Gaining a new view of what is happening around us, avoiding being influenced by negativity and toxic judgments, which can affect our existence, and make it difficult to relate to ourselves and others.
- Deepen aspects of the archetypal patterns that exist within us, to know how to deal with taboos and shadows that stagnate at the energetic level, preventing our inner light from illuminating us.
- Learn, through an experiential path, to offer our support to those close to us in both personal and professional spheres.
- Expand the listening skills, imagination, and courage that it takes to face a life that coincides with our inner desire, and that makes us healthy, free and happy men.

All this is achieved by observing oneself to correct oneself and take constructive action.
Because we can only change or improve what we notice. Self-observation will enable us to understand what is right to be and then do at a given time, with enormous benefits in daily life.

FEAR THE MOTHER OF ALL EMOTIONS

Anxiety, worry, and negative imagination are just some derivatives of the fear that very often drives our actions. All human beings are vulnerable to fear. How can we observe and transform it? Everyone has an interest in creating constructive actions and keeping up the immune defenses that are so valuable to one's well-being, so it is essential to address this issue and discover the tools to bring great benefit to one's life. Through 'empowerment, one learns to recognize the ballast of negative emotions, present in our existence, which generates all sorts of disasters and enables the acquisition of the abilities to transform everything into clean energy, for one's own benefit and for others.

SELF-SABOTAGE AND ITS DESTRUCTIVENESS IN DAILY LIFE

Self-sabotage is one of the activities in which human beings are unfortunately the highest experts. It is highly destructive and most individuals perform self-sabotage actions unknowingly, especially when we have to change to live a new way of dealing with our health.

How can we recognize this inner world that determines being a prey instead of a maker? Again through the method of self-observation, of the main dynamics that humans incur so that we can make a correction that brings great benefits.

NEEDS AND VALUES

We have grown up without having the basic elements of inner knowing. Unable mostly to recognize our own needs, often confused with those of someone else more or less close to us, we are unable to direct our actions so that the same needs are met. Values, these unknown or lost, are no longer the beacon of our lives, they have become watered down, polluted, leaving man without reference points, without an anchor ready to support him especially in times of difficulty. The new perception of our self allows the resurfacing of this precious forgotten inner world.

THE ART OF ASKING QUESTIONS: SOCRATES DOCET

As adults, one loses the power to ask questions nevertheless it remains invaluable for knowing, deepening, analyzing, reflecting to learn to be present to oneself, free thinkers instead of sleepy followers of someone or something. What is health? What is the economy? What is freedom? What makes me feel good? Acquiring this skill is of infinite help in everyday life.

ACT OR REACT, WHAT ARE THE EFFECTS?

Exploring the power of expectation, kindness and gratitude can help tremendously in managing personal and professional relationships. Acquiring better relationship management skills raises the level of relationships, leading to greater harmony and effectiveness.

WE ARE THE PROBLEM, WE ARE THE SOLUTION

In this statement the responsibility for our actions is revealed. But what are our actions generated by? What do we know about the uncontrolled river of thoughts, feelings and emotions that swirl within us and yet are the incontrovertible fuse of everything we put into being? It is essential to become aware that the process of creating reality follows an inside-out movement that will make a difference in one's life, forever.

MEA CULPA - THE GREAT REVERSAL

Mea Culpa is the formula for a responsibility that knows no bounds. In these two words lies the secret of boundless energy. Their meaning is that everything that happens, everything, depends on us and no one else in the entire universe. Hard words to accept in a time when the other is always guilty and we are victims. It is essential to question certainties and create a vacuum so that there is room to fill it with new virtuous habits that replace old harmful habits.

LANGUAGE AND ITS DECEPTION

The verb creates. Language is the manifestation of who we are; it should correspond to what we think and be preceded by coherent action. Instead the opposite happens, not only are we not in control of our thoughts and thus the words that follow but coherence rarely follows. This process in itself makes one dissatisfied, confused, and angry about the misalignment between being and doing that ensues. First, the fundamentals. Learn the new paradigm: being-doing-having-sharing.

TRANSURFING - LEARNING TRUE RESILIENCE

Reprogramming the destructive mind through a series of exercises is possible. Transurfing has an O.B. approach consisting of three main components: «how we think, how we fuel, how we move.» Deeply understanding the causes of one's successes and failures exponentially increases one's ability to replicate the conditions that allowed the inner power to unleash positive effects in our lives.

One understands how to navigate rough or murky waters and come out stronger. Resilience, lowering importance, internal and external intention are just some of the themes that will help us improve.

ACTING: ROLES AND IDENTITY

Gaining full awareness about the difference between who we are and the roles we play in society is of paramount importance. We are able to remain ourselves regardless of the «tasks» manifested in life, we learn detachment instead of identification, and we learn the need to return to our center. These are all fundamental to a harmonious existence, the antechamber of positive circumstances and events.

RELATIONSHIPS - AUTHENTICITY AND RECOGNITION

Man is constantly seeking approval and consensus, nagged by the fear of others' judgment and in a constant race to conform to the latest fashion/slogan/politician/influencer. He does not know himself and thus has lost the capacity for authentic, free and independent thinking. He has difficulty recognizing the positive in his fellow man and focuses attention almost predominantly on the negative aspects. New perceptions allows us the recovery of awareness about mirror play and deep wisdom that will bring great changes in relationship life.

THE DREAM AND HAPPINESS

The term dream has been abused in advertisements, talk shows, and language. Through Orthomolecular Biohacking we will have the total recovery of our deepest sense. Regaining this seventh sense, after the sixth, that is, intuition, is essential to access the dimension of governing one's own existence. Understanding what the process is for the realization of one's dreams and accessing the dimension of «creators of one's destiny» is a fundamental step in the life of every human being who wishes to use his or her talents, follow his or her divine plan and use life experience to elevate being and thus doing, consequent having to result in sharing, in a virtuous circle that improves exponentially.

Chapter 24
Intermittent fasting

«And when you fast, do not assume a melancholy air like the hypocrites, who disfigure their faces so that men may see that they fast. Verily I tell you, they have already received their reward. But you, when you fast, perfume your head and wash your face, so that people may not see that you fast, but only your Father who is in secret; and your Father, who sees in secret, will reward you.»

Jesus - Sermon on the Mount

Fasting is a healing technique that has its roots in the mists of time integrated into all mono- and polytheistic religions.

Muslims

Muslims fast in the month of Ramadan, the ninth in the lunar and sacred calendar, because the faithful belief that Muhammad received the revelation of the Quran from the archangel Gabriel during that period. It represents one of the five obligatory pillars for the Muslim faithful, and consists of abstaining from dawn to dusk from drinking, eating, smoking and engaging in sexual activities. The reason for fasting is self-control, and they believe that through this practice man's soul is freed from the chains of his bodily cravings. Fasting also makes one understand the value of God's gifts and thus allows one to be open to those in need, thus enticing the believer to pour out lazakat, or alms.

Christians

Christians fast on Ash Wednesday and Good Friday following a fast consisting of abstinence from meat every Friday of Lent.
The meaning of this fast is metonymy, or the spiritual transformation that brings man closer to God. One fasts not only by abstaining from food but also from everything that is addictive.

Jews

Jews fast 6 days in the year, the most important Yom Kippur, which occurs in the 10th month. This is a day of purification and atonement. The fast is intended to help the soul rise above physical needs and connect more directly with the divine. Fasting symbolizes humility and purification. The soul is elevated through denial of the physical body's typical comfort.

WHAT IS INTERMITTENT FASTING?

Intermittent fasting is an eating practice that involves periods of abstaining from food intake interspersed with periods of regular eating. There are several ways to practice intermittent fasting, but the most common are:

1. Fasting 16/8h: performs lipolytic action that is activated after at least 12 hours of consecutive fasting. This method involves a 16-hour fasting period and an 8-hour feeding window. Usually one chooses to do the fast overnight and only starts eating from the following morning, essentially moving breakfast to late morning (*brunch*, a combination of *breakfast* and *lunch*) During the feeding period it is important to maintain a balanced and healthy diet.
2. Fasting 20/24h: Basically this involves eating in the evening trying to spread the dinner meal out over a couple of hours and after dinner perhaps taking a nice walk while avoiding lying down with a full stomach. As a rule let at least a couple of hours pass before sleeping lying down.
3. OMAD (one meal day): that is, one meal every 23 hours. It lowers fat mass and increases lean mass by stabilizing insulin levels, increasing the release of Testosterone, Serotonin, GH. OMAD alone stimulates autophagy processes and activation of indigenous stem cell synthase. It stimulates autophagy of disintegrating (DNA fragments, waste, toxins, etc.) and potentially damaging (inflammaging) cells by increasing stem cell turnover that activates major healing processes. For example, it increases production of AMPKINases and Sirtuins. 5' AMP-activated protein kinase or AMPK or 5' adenosine monophosphate-activated protein kinase is an enzyme that plays a role in cellular energy homeostasis, mainly to activate the uptake and oxidation of glucose and fatty acids when cellular energy is low.
4. Alternate fasting: alternating days of fasting with days of regular diet. On the fasting day, a limited amount of food is consumed (usually around 500-600 calories) and an attempt is made to limit the consumption of carbohydrates and sugars.

5. Every other day fasting: in this case one could eat for 3 days, fast for a full day, resume eating for two more days and fast for the last day of the week.

Before starting intermittent fasting, it is important to consult a doctor or nutritionist to make sure it is suitable for your needs and health condition. In addition, during the fasting period it is important to drink plenty of water and limit coffee and tea consumption to avoid dehydration.

AUTOPHAGY

In 2016 Prof Yoshinori Ohsumi was awarded the Nobel Prize in Physiology or Medicine for his discoveries on the mechanisms of «autophagy.» Autophagy (self-eating) is a process by which cells selectively degrade and recycle cellular components.

Ohsumi's research has focused primarily on yeast, but he has also studied autophagy in plants. In fact, for the past two decades Professor Ohsumi has chosen to publish his work in The Plant Cell and Plant Physiology. You can see some of his contributions to the study of autophagy in plants here. Autophagy in cells cultured in tobacco suspension in response to sucrose starvation (1996). Y. Moriyasu and Y. Ohsumi. Plant Physiol. 111: 1233 - 1241. Foliar senescence and starvation-induced chlorosis are accelerated by fasting disruption of Arabidopsis autophagy (2002). Hideki Hanaoka, Takeshi Noda, Yumiko Shirano, Tomohiko Kato, Hiroaki Hayashi, Daisuke Shibata, Satoshi Tabata, and Yoshinori Ohsumi. Plant Physiol. 129: 1181 - 1193.

The processing of ATG8, ubiquitin-like proteins and their deconjugation by ATG4 are essential for plant autophagy (2004). Kohki Yoshimoto, Hideki Hanaoka, Shusei Sato, Tomohiko Kato, Satoshi Tabata, Takeshi Noda, and Yoshinori Ohsumi. Plant Cell 16: 2967 - 2983.

An Arabidopsis homolog of the yeast ATG6/VPS30 is essential for pollen germination (2007). Yuki Fujiki, Kohki Yoshimoto, and Yoshinori Ohsumi. Plant Physiol. 143: 1132 - 1139.

Localized fluorescent protein mobilization of rubisco and chloroplast stroma in the vacuole by an autophagy-dependent process of the ATG gene (2008). Hiroyuki Ishida, Kohki Yoshimoto, Masanori Izumi, Daniel Reisen, Yuichi Yano, Amane Makino, Yoshinori Ohsumi, Maureen R. Hanson, and Tadahiko Mae. Plant Physiol. 148: 142 - 155.

Autophagy plays a role in chloroplast degradation during senescence in individually darkened leaves (2009). Shinya Wada, Hiroyuki Ishida, Masanori Izumi, Kohki Yoshimoto, Yoshinori Ohsumi, Tadahiko Mae, and Amane Makino. Plant Physiol. 149: 885 - 893.
Autophagy negatively regulates cell death by controlling NPR1-dependent salicylic acid signaling during senescence and innate immune response in Arabidopsis (2009). Kohki Yoshimoto, Yusuke Jikumaru, Yuji Kamiya, Miyako Kusano, Chiara Consonni, Ralph Panstruga, Yoshinori Ohsumi, and Ken Shirasu. Plant Cell 21: 2914 - 2927. Highly oxidized peroxisomes are selectively degraded by autophagy in Arabidopsis (2013). Michitaro Shibata, Kazusato Oikawa, Kohki Yoshimoto, Maki Kondo, Shoji Mano, Kenji Yamada, Makoto Hayashi, Wataru Sakamoto, Yoshinori Ohsumi, and Mikio Nishimura. Plant Cell 25: 4967 - 4983.
Professor Ohsumi's research is also discussed in the article Teaching Tools in Plant Biology «The End: Senescence and Cell Death.»

16/24 HYDRO KETOGENIC/AUTOPHAGY PRE-OMAD DIET USED BY A SENIOR MULTISPORT ATHLETE (A.P.).

Breakfast
- Apple cider vinegar 2 tablespoons
- Green tea with moringa or oolong, matcha, no sweetener, with light water
- Either: Bresaola 50 gr, turkey breast, tuna 50 gr, organic omelet (omelet with three whites and half of a yolk), or 4 hard-boiled eggs without the yolk + 2 cakes of puffed rice or quinoa and amaranth
- Use of tea is instrumental in stimulating detox and anorectic processes. Useful to consume at least 2 liters throughout the day (4 bs x 2 lt of tea)

Mid-morning
- Berries 1 teacup (blueberries, currants, etc.)

Lunch
- Raw and/or cooked green leafy vegetables, 180g and seasoned only with lemon and granulated dijon mustard or classic mustard;
- Choice of: two hamburger red meat or turkey or skinless chicken 180, white fish 300g (tuna also desired though not white fish), 3 white and 1/2 red eggs (organic omelet), or every 3 days casein-free cheese (see list)

Mid-afternoon
- A fruit

Dinner
- Brown rice, quinoa, or amaranthus 50 gr (either lunch or dinner)

NB: If you were to eat refined carbohydrates, choose unrefined pasta or rice, and take 1 psyllium gel in 2 glasses of water
- Vegetable puree;
- Raw or cooked green vegetables 200 g
- One of the other alternatives not consumed at lunch

Before bedtime
- 3 almonds + 1 teaspoon pine nuts

If one is hungry during the day: carrots, celery, cooked fennel in unlimited quantities. Raw vegetables, coffee, bread, pizza, sweets, sugar and any kind of tea other than green or oolong are to be excluded at this stage. Only 18C steel pots should be used, without Chromium and without Nickel or Cobalt; no nonstick pans, if anything a drop of oil to be dabbed on later with paper.

OMAD FASTING FOR MEN, FOLLOWED BY SENIOR MULTISPORT ATHLETE A.P.

Breakfast
- Apple cider vinegar 2 tablespoons;
- Green tea with moringa or oolong tea, macha, no sweetener, with light water e.g. St. Anne's (4-6 cups over the morning).

Mid-morning and afternoon
- 3-4 olives and 1 coffee cup of Chia seeds + 1 coffee cup of coffee (almonds, cashews, pine nuts, macadamia nuts, pistachios) + 1 teacup full of blueberries, raspberries, currants + 2 rice cakes or quinoa or amaranth;

Dinner
- 50 g corn or rice pasta (garlic and oil or added cooked vegetables or mushrooms);

→

- Cooked green leafy vegetables, 100-150 g seasoned with lemon or apple cider vinegar and a teaspoon of granular or mustard and 1 teaspoon of EVO oil.
- Choice of: veal cutlet 200 gr, roast beef, skinless turkey or chicken 200 gr, white fish 300gr (if desired also tuna though not white fish)
- 3 white and 1/2 red eggs (organic omelet), or every 3 days casein-free cheese like tofu.

OMAD FASTING FOR WOMEN, DIETARY REGIMEN FOLLOWED BY SENIOR FEMALE ATHLETE S.S.

Breakfast

- Apple cider vinegar 2 tablespoons
- Green tea with moringa or oolong tea, macha, no sweetener, with light water (4-6 cups over the morning)

Mid-morning and afternoon

- 3 -4 olives and a coffee cup espresso of Chia seeds + 1 coffee cup portion (espresso) (almonds, cashews, pine nuts, macadamia nuts, pistachios) + 1 teacup full of blueberries, blackberries, raspberries, currants + 2 rice cakes or quinoa or amaranth
- Green tea with moringa or oolong tea, macha, no sweetener, with light water (4 cups within the first afternoon)

Dinner

- 50 g corn or rice pasta (garlic and oil or added cooked vegetables or mushrooms)
- Green leafy vegetables (raw) and/or cooked, 150-180 g seasoned with lemon and a teaspoon of granular or classic mustard and 1 tsp. oil
- Choice of: veal cutlets 150, gr roast beef or skinless turkey or chicken 180 gr, white fish 300g (wanting also tuna though not white fish) - 3 white and 1/2 red eggs (organic omelet), or every 3 days casein-free cheese like tofu.

Chapter 25

The Man Who Came in from the Cold

«What is cold gets warm, what is hot gets cold, wet gets dry, dry gets wet.»
Heraclitus

Immersing oneself in cold water is a practice quite in vogue in the martial arts and, from a very young age, before I reached the much coveted black belt my Karate Master Wadoryu initiated me into an initiatory practice that I want to share with you since it promises to generate several benefits to the body. This is not entirely new since it seems to have existed for millennia; however, today it is possible to practice it making use of state-of-the-art techniques that can keep the parameters in check body and to ensure safe conduct.

In an OB (Orthomolecular Biohacking) program, it is important to dwell on initiatory mountain practices and related purification rituals, often implemented along with other ascetic exercises such as sleep deprivation and strict fasting. In Shinto, the practice of Misogi means meditation under the waterfall and bathing in very cold or icy water. The purpose of this technique is to purify oneself of sins and defilements that the body has been subjected to. There are similarities with the ancient Greek practice of LUSTRATIO, a true ceremony of bodily purification.

In Buddhism, meditation under the waterfall is called Takigyō. This word means «to stand under the waterfall.» The second term is Takishugyō 滝修行, this practice means «The hard practice under the waterfall» which consists of a week-long exercise where, three times a day, one meditates under the jets of water coming down from the waterfall.

Winter ascetic practices are called Kangyō, which means «Hard Winter Practices.» The tradition of this ritual goes back to the Shinto legend of the deity Izanami no Mikoto, who purified himself at sea after Having crossed

Yomi, the realm of the dead. For the ritual, a kind of light white summer kimono called yukata 浴衣 is used.
In the Land of the Rising Sun, the color white is the color of death and mourning; in the Takigyō ritual, one «ritually dies» and is cleansed of sins and bad influences by cold water and then is reborn. The Takigyō Rite can be performed under any waterfall suitable for this purpose; however, there are (considered sacred specific ones) in Japan that are specifically used by monks for this cathartic ritual.
Waterfall meditation not only has a religious or ascetic character, but is often practiced in Japanese Martial Arts such as Karate, Ninjutsu or Aikidō to harden and strengthen the body and mind. Karate masters such as Jitsumi Gōgenamaguchi or Masatatsu Oyama, Toyama were famous for their kime', which they developed under the waterfall by performing Sanshin kata with the correct Ibuki breathing technique.
Personally as a martial arts practitioner and as a student of Master Toyama, I have had the opportunity to approach and practice these extreme workouts under waterfalls, on freshly fallen snow at high altitude. This process referred to in electrology as «Negatization» is capable of enhancing the immune system and improving adaptogenic abilities to the environment in which we must integrate. Negatization is the way in which our mitochondria, true cellular powerhouses, recharge our meridian energy pathways, restoring the metabolic pathways essential for life to flow fluidly through our bodies.
Also in the Shingon Buddhist school, but especially in Shugendō, Takigyō is often practiced throughout the year, sometimes at night when the moon is full. Many Yamabushi make a pilgrimage specifically to the areas of Mount Ontake, the Kii Mountains or Mount Yoshino to practice Takigyō. Now there are different methods and techniques as well as Deities and prayers that you have to pay attention to in Takigyō. In Shintoism you worship various Kami in the forests and ask them for purification.
«Harae Tamae Kiyomi Tamae Rokon Shojo»: this mantric phrase asks the Kami to wash away the impurity of the six senses and purify the mind. However, the best known Buddhist form is the transformation into Fudō Myō and the invocation of the Fudō Mantra. The waterfall represents a direct connection between the Taizokai universe and the material world of Kongokai.
When the initiate goes under the waterfall using various techniques, he visualizes the syllable seed of Fudō Myō and through the correct use of Sanmitsu or Kuji In and Kuji kiri, the ascetic becomes Fudō Myō himself,

empties himself of all his negative charge and is recharged with clean energy. Takigyō practice should be regarded not only as protection, asceticism, religious practice, breathing and resilience, but also as integration with nature. However, it is also a very hard and rigid practice that one should never undertake alone without experience or the proper teacher. If one does not know the spiritual techniques and Mudras behind it, Takigyo remains nothing more than a cold shower. The pressure of the water and the negatively charged ions in the water massage the Crown Chakra located outside our physical body above the head. Every waterfall and every place has a different surrounding aura, and the ascetic also feels different experiences during his or her practice. Once again, however, I would like to warn that many people who go under a waterfall alone without knowing the practice should never underestimate the power and dangers inherent in the Energies of Nature.

For us in the West, cold water therapy, also known as Cold hydrotherapy involves using water at less than 15°C to treat medical conditions or stimulate positive health effects. It is usually done by immersing in a tub filled with water, but there are different techniques. There would be several benefits of practicing cold water therapy, including improved blood circulation and quality of sleep, mitochondrial activation, that is, increased energy levels, and reduced body inflammation. Years ago, when I was following Djokovic, I was considered a Martian because as his personal physician, I recommended that he soak in cold water for short periods after training, finding a huge reduction in muscle and injury pain. Needless to say, 10 years later, the use of cryotherapy with ice water immersion baths have become a simple routine in the practice of many sports.

Cold water causes vasoconstriction, reducing blood flow in a given section of the body. Just think of applying ice to a contusion or wound to reduce swelling and inflammation. To facilitate muscle recovery, ice water therapy can be supplemented by performing stretching or active recovery exercises directly at low temperature. With Djokovic we have been able to achieve much faster post-workout recovery times by using cold water at a temperature of about 10°C, thus helping the body to lower its temperature much faster than simply active rest in a cool environment. We verified, with Nole Djokovic, therefore, the use after intense training of ice water therapy given it is done by soaking the entire body in the liquid and not just the wrists under the cold jet as our grandparents taught is superior.

As a psychologist, as well as a physician, I also want to report an alleviation of depression symptoms. This is not to argue that cold water can be a cure

for conditions of mental distress; however, some studies suggest cold open water swimming to alleviate depressive symptoms and a recent new research, published in the British Medical Journal Case Reports, reinforces this view and adds that cold open water swimming may be an even more efficacious treatment.
The study, led by Chris van Tulleken of University College London and two scientists from the University of Portsmouth, looked at the experience of a 24-year-old woman with major depressive disorder and anxiety. The woman had been in therapy since she was 17 but, at the time she became a mother, she tried hard to find a way to counter depression without using medication. The patient therefore began regular open-water swimming sessions under the supervision of the same researchers. The latter noticed an immediate improvement in her mood after each swim. As she continued with these sessions, the woman gradually managed to decrease the amounts of medication until she stopped them.
Researchers therefore began to suspect that the beneficial cause lay in cold water immersion. Indeed, this practice causes a stress response through a series of physiological and hormonal reactions, reactions that have been evolving in the human body for millions of years. By swimming regularly in cold water, the body learns to gradually reduce this chronic stress response but at the same time also reduces symptoms related to anxiety and depression.

Sources and insights

- *Cold water swimming might ease depression (IA)*
- *Open water swimming as a treatment for major depressive disorder - van Tulleken et al. 2018 - BMJ Case Reports (DOI: 10.1136/bcr-2018-225007) (IA)*

Cold water therapy stimulates by strengthening the immune system. A Dutch study divided participants into two groups and then exposed them to a bacterial infection. One was asked to practice meditation techniques, deep breathing and cold water immersion, while the other was not. In the end, people part of the first would develop fewer symptoms and their bodies produced more anti-inflammatory chemicals and fewer pro-inflammatory cytokines in response to the infection.

Although more research is needed to determine whether cold water therapy can help with weight loss, some studies have shown that it can speed up the metabolic rate and thus the rate at which the body uses energy and burns calories.

How to practice cold water therapy:

If you want to try cold water therapy for the first time, it is necessary to proceed in small steps.

Alternate hot and cold showers.

Start the shower with lukewarm water and, after a few minutes, gradually lower the temperature.

Take a cold shower immediately after exercising.

Fill a bathtub with water, adding ice until the temperature is between 10°C and 15°C, then soak for 10 to 15 minutes.

Take a short swim in cold water.

How to do cold water therapy safely

Talk to your doctor first. Because cold water immersion affects blood pressure, heart rate and circulation, it can cause severe cardiac stress. Before practicing it, therefore, it is essential to talk to your doctor and assess any risks with him or her, in relation to your baseline health status.

Don't do it alone the first time. Since it is impossible to know your body's reactions to the impact of intense cold, the first few times you practice cold water therapy it would be best to do so by having a person nearby who can intervene in case of the onset of discomfort or problems of various kinds. By practicing cold water therapy, your body temperature may continue to drop even after you get out of the water, increasing the risk of hypothermia. Once finished, therefore, it is essential to try to warm up instantly by removing wet clothing and replacing it with dry, warm clothing, starting with the upper body. At this point, to help the body return to optimal temperature, you can walk to raise your body temperature, drink a hot drink, and eat something sweet, as sugar raises body temperature.

In conclusion, if you want to practice cold therapy, do so only after consulting an experienced physician.

Chapter 26

Awakening of dormant muscle fibers: ten thousand sissy squats/day, facilitated with elastic binds

---

«The good and the wise lead quiet lives» [...not always!].

Euripides [challenged by Adolfo Panfili].

Why embark on this path? Basically, to get sick less, take fewer medications and, with a little luck that never hurts, live long and feel better, paraphrasing the recommendations of multiple Nobel laureate and my teacher of life and science Professor Linus Pauling (L. Pauling. *How to live longer and feel better*, Paper Newton Book). I personally practice daily deadlift squats on a piece of equipment I designed and built (a.panfili@aimo.it), known as the sissy squat machine using rubber bands tied to a hook that allows for a high number of repetitions and stimulates the activation of dormant muscle fibers that are not routinely used when performing submaximal efforts and for low numbers of repetitions.

My colleague and friend Prof. Conconi, a true sportsman and practitioner, implemented an interesting project to control type 2 diabetes in the province of Ferrara. That project was based on having patients practice a low-impact daily sports activity, such as walking at a brisk pace for 10,000 steps a day, or covering a total distance of 5 km. At the same time, these patients were prescribed a low-calorie diet of 1200 kcal/day for women and 1500 kcal/day for men. The results were excellent: less medication and more health. In addition, performing daily physical activity was associated with a 27% decrease in mortality risk. Currently, 60 minutes of moderate activity on most days of the week. Such a small sacrifice is possible for most of you readers. Any type of physical activity for sedentary individuals represents an important opportunity to decrease mortality risk (*Archives of Internal Medicine*, 2007, 167: 2453-60). Activating slumbering muscle fibers (muscle sleeping fibers) with long duration exercise at increasing intensity is only possible with the aid of facilitators of the execution of the gesture. In this case I use elastic bands that allow physical exertion to continue well beyond the threshold of muscle acidosis, awakening the sleeping fibers to be enlisted in the totalizing movement. Therefore, using more cells to burn more fat and releasing greater amounts of adaptive hormones to feel better. Obviously, this mode must be achieved progressively and requires perfect execution of the movement. The program, in addition to the execution of the fateful 1000 Sissy Squats with elastic bands, also provides tips to increase movement opportunities and increase MB:

FIT-EASY PROGRAM

- Use the stairs, even for a few floors, instead of using the elevator;
- limit car use, perhaps parking farther from the destination to walk some of the route, or get off the bus a stop earlier, or use a bicycle;
- avoid sitting too long;
- use the cell phone, intercom, or remote controls as little as possible and try to move around to request something or deliver it;
- doing gardening (even if only on the terrace) and household chores while avoiding the use of small appliances (electric broom, cheese grater, electric toothbrush...);
- play with your children by participating in traditional movement games (flag stealing, four cantons, hide-and-seek...).

Summary of energy cost values measured in various physical activities

Activities	Kcal/h in 50 kg subject	Kcal/h in 70 kg subject	Kcal/h in subject from 90 kg
Archery	150 - 200	210 - 280	270 - 360
Basketball	150 - 600	280 - 630	360 - 810
Billiards	125	175	225
Bowling	100 - 200	140 - 280	180 - 360
Boxing	400 - 650	560 - 910	720 - 1170
Canoeing/Rowing	150 - 400	210 - 560	270 - 720
Cycling	150 - 400	210 - 560	270 - 720
Sissy squat vacuum with elastic bands	150 - 400	210 - 560	270 - 720
Dance	150 - 350	210 - 490	270 - 630
Aerobics	200 - 500	280 - 700	360 - 900
Fencing	300 - 500	420 - 700	540 - 900
Valtraining	450 - 650	560 - 910	720 - 1170
Golf	100 - 150	140 - 210	180 - 270
Handball	400 - 600	560 - 840	720 - 1080
Riding	150 - 400	210 - 560	270 - 720
Mountaineering	150 - 500	350 - 700	450 - 900
Takigyo	400 - 650	600 - 1000	800 - 1200

Chapter 27

Hypoxic workout to empower mithocondria: my experience with Djokovic

"You can choose to live or to die. Every minutes is a choice to breathe or not to breathe. To be or not to be".

Chuck Palahniuk

Hypoxia is the condition where there is a lower than the normal oxygen concentration in the arterial blood. It happens when there is an interruption of the normal mithocondrial respiratory chain due to breathing disorders and therefore it can be the result of respiratory inadequacy. Covid infection was able to decrease breathing exchange along the alveoli's mucosa creating sudden low grading of oxygen saturation with all the consequences that we have experienced during this epidemia. The last years, the response of the human cells, tissues and body to either induced or innate hypoxia has attracted a lot of attention from the scientific community. In 2019 nobel prize in physiology or medicine was awarded jointly to William G. Kaelin Jr, Sir Peter J. Ratcliffe and Gregg L. Semenza "for their discoveries of how cells sense and adapt to oxygen avai-lability."

They identified molecular machinery that regulates the activity of genes in response to varying levels of oxygen that of course will influence the cell redox potential conditioning TP Protein 53 (inhibitor oncogene see Chapter 28).

In parallel to their research, further studies on the effect of the intermittent hypoxia was intensified during the last 5 years all around the world. The use of the so-called intermittent hypoxia therapy (IHT) in athletic and mi-litary practices as well as medical applications for prevention and treat-ment of various diseases has gained interest among the scientific community and has shed light to the beneficial potential of the technology.

WHAT IS THE PRIMARY BIOLOGICAL EFFECT OF INTERMITTENT HYPOXIA?

The compensatory nature of the effect of the Intermittent Hypoxia on the human cells and consequently on the human tissues seems to be a complex issue. A lot of different mechanisms are modulated by intermittent hypoxia such as (but not limited to):

- Downregulation of reactive oxygen (ROS) and nitrogen (RNS) species
- Expression of hypoxia responsive genes including some for erythropoietin and growth factors
- Control of mitochondrial quality

These mechanisms are often interlinked and the basic research is focusing on exploring further their role to disease and its prevention, its treatment and even its healing

HOW IS HYPOXIC THERAPY DONE?

It involves breathing in hypoxic (low oxygen) air with intervals of hyperoxic (high oxygen) air. Normoxic (normal oxygen concentration) phases can replace the hyperoxic phases, but are generally less efficient, since the restoration of the normal Sp02 levels takes longer and the effect of the succesive hypoxic phase is decreased. The patient quietly inhales the air mixture supplied by the precisely controlled unit through a mask.

HYPOXIC MITHOCONDRIAL BOOSTER

IHT significantly improves the control of mitochondrial quality, which is regulated by balance between the biogenesis -birth of new- and autophagic destruction -death of old- of mitochondria. In simpler words, a self imposed quality control is achieved by the establishment of fine balance between the elimination of damaged and dysfunctional mitochondria and the generation of new and "healthy" mitochondria.

Data sources and study selection: A systematic search was conducted to capture all LLTH studies with a matched normoxic (control) training group and the assessment of performance under normoxic conditions. Studies were excluded if no training was completed during the hypoxic exposures, or if these exposures exceeded 3 h per day. Four electronic databases were searched (PubMed, SPORTDiscus, EMBASE and Web of Science) during August 2013, and these searches were supplemented by additional manual searches until December 2013.

Results: After the electronic and manual searches, 40 papers were deemed to meet the inclusion criteria, representing 31 separate studies. Within these 31 studies, four types of LLTH were identified:
1) Continuos low-intensity training in hypoxia (CHT, n = 16),
2) Interval hypoxic training (IHT, n = 4),
3) Repeated sprint training in hypoxia (RSH, n = 3) and
4) Resistence training in hypoxia (RTH, n = 4). Four studies also used a combination of CHT and IHT.
The majority of studies reported no difference in normoxic performance between the hypoxic and normoxic training groups (n = 19), while nine reported greater improvements in the hypoxic group and three reported poorer outcomes compared with the control group. Selection of training intensity (including matching relative or absolute intensity between normoxic and hypoxic groups) was identified as a key factor in mediating the subsequent normoxic performance outcomes. Five studies included some form of normoxic training for the hypoxic group and 14 studies assessed performance outcomes not specific to the training intensity/modality completed during the training intervention.
Conclusion: Four modes of LLTH are identified in the current literature (CHT, IHT, RSH and RTH), with training mode and intensity appearing to be key factors in mediating subsequent performance responses in normoxia. Improvements in normoxic performance appear most likely following high-intensity, short-term and intermittent training (e.g., IHT, RSH). LLTH programmes should carefully apply the principles of training and testing specificity and include some high-intensity training in normoxia. For RTH, it is unclear whether the associated adaptations are greater than those of traditional (maximal) resistance training programmes.

IHT(Interval Hipoxic Training) enhances athletic performances and do not adversely affect immune function in middle/- long distance runners(Won-Sang Jung et al. Int J Environ Res Public Health. 2020)

This study evaluated the effects of intermittent interval training in hypoxic conditions for six weeks compared with normoxic conditions, on hemodynamic function, autonomic nervous system (ANS) function, immune function, and athletic performance in middle- and long-distance runners. Twenty athletes were divided into normoxic training (normoxic training group (NTG); n = 10; residing and training at sea level) and hypoxic training (hypoxic training group (HTG); n = 10; residing at sea level but training in 526-mmHg hypobaric hypoxia) groups. All dependent variables were measured before, and after, training. The training frequency was 90 min, 3 d per week for six weeks. Body composition showed no significant difference between the two groups. However, the HTG showed more significantly improved athletic performance (e.g., maximal oxygen uptake). The hemodynamic function (e.g., oxygen uptake, oxygen pulse, and cardiac output) during submaximal exercise and ANS function (e.g., standard deviation and root mean square of successive differences, high frequency, and low/high frequency) improved more in the HTG. Immune function parameters were stable within the normal range before and after training in both groups. Therefore, hypoxic training was more effective in enhancing athletic performance, and improving hemodynamic and ANS function; further, it did not adversely affect immune function in competitive runners.

Chapter 28

Sleep to lose weight: sleepslimming

«Life and dreams are sheets of the same book. To read them in order is to live, to flip through them at random is to dream.»

Arthur Schopenhauer

During sleep, you lose weight. So those suffering from sleep disorders may encounter more difficulties in maintaining weight and/or slimming down.

Granted that insomnia is an extremely serious problem that needs to be addressed by experienced medical personnel, you can in the meantime try to solve the problem by following some simple behavioral rules such as the following:

SLEEP TIPS.

Go to bed at night and get up in the morning always at the same time;

Do not lie down unless you are sleepy;

Sleep only the number of hours sufficient to feel rested;

Make sure the bedroom has a comfortable temperature (about 18°C), is quiet and dark;

Don't stay in bed if, after thirty minutes you still haven't gotten to sleep... Devote yourself to your workout session and then take a nice hot bath of about twenty minutes with water at 38 °C diluted with 300 g of disodium bicarbonate and get ready to... dream;

Avoid afternoon naps or limit it to half an hour at most;

Avoid evening meals that are too large, but do not go to bed hungry;

Listen to relaxing music (432 hz) or read-these are habits that can promote a good night's rest;

In the afternoon and evening, avoid exciting substances such as the caffeine or nicotine;

Once you are in bed, do not face any discussions; if you have to pay your mortgage that is due and you are in the red in the bank, staying up all night will certainly not replenish your bank account;

Pray or meditate: it helps to soothe the body, mind and soul;

Do not drink alcohol: it leads to fragmentation of sleep and the make restless;

Do not engage in particularly strenuous physical activity in the evening before bedtime;

Half an hour before bedtime, take 50 drops in hot water of the following cocktail of mother tinctures that you will have prepared by your trusted pharmacist or herbalist: Valerian Officinalis TM 40% + Passiflora Incarnata TM 20% + Lupulus TM 20% + Lemon Balm Officinalis TM 20% + 68% vol Ethanolum.

Chapter 29
Slimming down by drinking: drink-slimming

«Any complicated phenomenon can be explained through simple scientific principles.»
Linus Pauling

Remember to drink the famous 2 liters of water a day, and let it be water and nothing else: there are no drinks in nature, much less commercially, that can match it. For scientific objectivity, however, it is appropriate to point out that, in fact, drinking too much water during a cross-country athletic race, such as a marathon, can cause serious damage to the body, just like drinking too little water. This is revealed by a study published in the prestigious New England Journal of Medicine (NEJM).

According to Tom Derderian, author of a book on the history of the ancient and prestigious Boston Marathon, marathon runners were once a kind of test pilots of the human body, pushing the limits by running as no one had done until then. Currently, the marathon is a reasonably safe sport with less than one death per 50,000 participants. Contrary to what one might assume, in the case of the marathon, deaths are not solely attributable to cardiovascular causes: conditions such as rhabdomyolysis (destruction of muscle tissue) and other hydration-related conditions also play a role.

Benjamin Levine, a cardiologist at the University of Texas Southwestern Medical Center, and Paul Thompson, director of the Preventive Cardiology Program, Division of Preventive Cardiology at Hartford Hospital in Connecticut, authors of the study, found that marathon runners who drink too much water during a race are at risk of developing hyponatremia, a condition characterized by sodium deficiency in the body that can cause damage such as apathy, disorientation, seizures and respiratory crisis.

However, the risk would be less for professional athletes, Levine explains,

«Marathon runners who go at high speeds to win races also have less time to drink along the way. Instead, those who participate in races in a non-competitive spirit tend to stop at every refreshment point along the way and drink large amounts of water. This, over the course of a race that lasts hours, leads them to 'dilute' themselves.» The most popular energy drinks used by athletes also do not always have sodium percentages sufficient to replenish the mineral loss incurred during prolonged exertion.

ENRICHED WATERS OR ALCHEMICAL DRINKS?

Water is an inalienable good, a right for everyone, often denied to most of humanity, which of this «transparent gold» (see Authors' Water the Transparent Gold, Macropost, 1998) laments the shortage. Replacing it with fruit juices or soft drinks is an ill-advised choice. At most, to vary its taste, one can add a few squeezed half lemons to the water, which will surely make it more thirst-quenching.

Be very careful with carbonated and caffeinated soft drinks. Caffeine in some soft drinks, such as cola, for example, would provide no contribution to the taste of the soft drink but, according to some experts, is intended to be addictive in consumers (International Appetite, Jan. 2007, Australia).

Russel Keast and Lynn Riddella of Deakin University in Melbourne, following various tests on about 30 20-year-olds, have shown, according to the data collected, that adding caffeine to soft drinks does not confer an appreciable improvement in taste; on the contrary, it can have dangerous effects on health in that creating addiction increases the risk of obesity due to the high amounts of sugar that characterize soft drinks.

The study also shows that there is no laboratory evidence to confirm what the companies that produce soft drinks such as cola claim, namely that caffeine would serve to impart a distinctive bouquet to soft drinks, since no test participant was able to detect the caffeine taste in the soft drinks tasted. At this point the question arises: why add caffeine to soft drinks? The caffeine contained in 500 ml of cola is sufficient to trigger a reaction at the level of the nervous system such that the drink is addictive.

There is a scientifically established relationship between the excessive consumption of soft drinks and the onset of obesity. In this regard, the Australian study illustrates that in children who drink sugary soft drinks also containing caffeine, an addiction could be triggered, and as soon as the effect of caffeine wears off, the little one is compulsively driven to take the drink again.

However, it is good not to overdo sugary drinks as their inordinate consumption contributes heavily to the establishment of obesity and consequently to the onset of type 2 diabetes and cardiovascular disease. Caffeine is an aroma belonging to a group of compounds found naturally in more than 60 plant species. The stimulant effects of caffeine vary from person to person and according to other factors such as age, weight, type of physical activity, and time of day when through a food or drink the substance is consumed. Caffeine has been an ingredient in cola drinks since their introduction over a hundred years ago. The amount of caffeine in cola drinks is very low, particularly when compared to other beverages (coffee, coffee liquor, tea): one-fourth to one-third less than, for example, coffee and tea. Useful instead are enrichments of amino acid, vitamin and minerals to water, as long as the organoleptic characters of the primitive water are respected.

THE PRINCIPLES ANTI-DEHYDRATION

Here are a series of wise tips for learning how to replenish yourself with the beneficial fluid every day:

- In the morning as soon as you wake up, drink two glasses of water;
- Always carry a bottle of water with you;
- Keep a good supply of water in the refrigerator;
- Replace coffee with green tea or herbal teas (dandelion is excellent, draining without dehydrating);
- Always drink in small sips, especially during meals;
- before sitting at the table, drink two full glasses of water: you will eat half, and have less hunger;
- Choose, whenever possible, soups and liquid foods instead of solid dishes;
- Eat at least 5 portions of vegetables a day;
- during sports activity, drink frequently to replenish the Fluid loss;
- if you walk or run or ride a bike, buy a «camel bag» or a simple water bottle at a sporting goods store;
- sip room temperature water whenever hunger arises, perhaps with a straw to activate the atavistic sucking reflex, which appears to stimulate the release of a rewarding neurotransmitter called dopamine.

Source:Altro Consumo

ACQUE MINERALI: DESCRIZIONE E RISULTATI DEL TEST								
MARCA e Denominazione in etichetta	Sorgente		Contenitore	Etichette	Residuo fisso mg/l	Sodio mg/l	Nitrati	Composizione caratteristiche principali
	Comune	altitudine						
Minimamente mineralizzate (residuo non superiore a 50 mg/l)								
MERANO S. VIGILIO oligominerale + CO_2	BZ	1540 m	vetro	★	20 ○	2.2 ○	○	basso tenore di sodio
NORDA DAGGIO min. mineralizzata	CO	558 m	vetro	★	48 ○	1.8 ○	○	basso tenore di sodio
PLOSE oligominerale	BZ	1830 m	vetro	★	16 ○	1.0 ○	○	basso tenore di sodio
S. BERNARDO oligominerale	CN	1000 m	/	★	40 ○	0.6 ○	○	basso tenore di sodio, cloruri solfati
Oligominerali (residuo compreso tra 50 e 500 mg/l)								
CINTOIA oligominerale	PI	400 m	tetrabrik	★	300 ○	7.7 ○	○	
CINZIA oligominerale	PS	801 m	tetrabrik	★	295 ○	9.8 ○	○	
CRODO LIESEL + CO_2	NO	510 m	PET	★	215 ○	4.7 ○	○	ricca di solfati
FABIA oligominerale	TR	330 m	PVC	□	430 ○	12.6 ○	★/□	
FIUGGI oligominerale	FR	590 m	vetro	★	115 ○	6.5 ○	★	
FONTE GAJUM oligominerale + CO_2	CO	481 m	vetro	★	265 ○	0.7 ○	★	basso tenore di sodio
FONTE GUIZZA minerale + CO_2	VE	20 m	PET	★	290 ○	4.5 ○	○	ricca di solfati
FONTENOVA minerale + CO_2	PR	447 m	vetro	★	125 ○	5.0 ○	○	
FRIDA oligominerale	VA	271 m	PET	★	225 ○	4.9 ○	□	basso tenore di sodio, tenore un po' troppo elevato di nitrati
GOCCIA DI CARNIA oligomin. + CO_2	UD	1370 m	vetro	★	85 ○	1.5 ○	○	basso tenore di sodio
LEVISSIMA oligominerale + CO_2	SO	1848 m	PET	★	60 ○	1.3 ○	○	ricca di solfati. basso tenore di sodio
LORA RECOARO minerale + CO_2	VI	800 m	PET	★	160 ○	0.5 ○	○/★	
MANGIATORELLA oligominerale	RC	1200 m	tetrabrik	★	55 ○	8.7 ○	○/★	
PANNA oligominerale	FI	292 m	vetro	★	135 ○	6.5 ○	○	
PINETA oligominerale + CO_2	BG	700 m	vetro	★	190 ○	0.4 ○	○	basso tenore di sodio
S. ANTONIO oligominerale + CO_2	CO	313 m	vetro	★	280 ○	3.9 ○	★	basso tenore di sodio
S. BENEDETTO minerale + CO_2	VE	20 m	PET	★	250 ○	3.8 ○	○	basso tenore di sodio
S. CROCE oligominerale	AQ	800 m	PET	★	200 ○	4.4 ○	○	basso tenore di sodio
S. GIORGIO minerale + CO_2	CA	400 m	vetro	□	250 ○	45.5 □	○	ricca di sodio, solfati, cloruri
S.STEFANO oligominerale + CO_2	SA	55 m	vetro	★	210 ○	4.1 ○	○	basso tenore di sodio
VALLECHIARA oligominerale + CO_2	SV	398 m	vetro	★	105 ○	4.3 ○	○	basso tenore di sodio
VERA oligominerale + CO_2	PD	60 m	PET	★	170 ○	2.2 ○	○	basso tenore di sodio
Medio minerali (residuo compreso tra 500 e 1500 mg/l)								
ACQUA DELLA MADONNA minerale	NA	6 m	vetro	★	865 ★	36 □	○/★	ricca di sodio, cloruri
BOARIO minerale + CO_2	BS	217 m	PET	★	860 ★	11.7 ○	★	forte tenore di solfati, non adatta ad un uso quotidiano
GAUDIANELLO minerale + CO_2	PZ	640 m	vetro	★	1400 □	119 □	★	acqua dura, ricca di sodio e solfati
LAVAREDO minerale + CO_2	BZ	271 m	vetro	★	1490 □	2.1 ○	○	forte tenore di solfati, non adatta ad un uso quotidiano
POZZILLO minerale + CO_2	CT	12 m	vetro	★	1460 □	196 □	□	tenore un pò troppo elevato di nitrati
PRACASTELLO minerale + CO_2	BG	358 m	vetro	★	935 ★	26.3 ★	○	forte tenore di solfati, non adatta ad un uso quotidiano
SACRAMORA minerale	FO	2 m	vetro	★	585 ★	32.7★/□	★/□	ricca di sodio, solfati, cloruri
S. ANDREA minerale + CO_2	PR	85 m	vetro	★	585 ★	85 □	○	ricca di sodio, solfati, cloruri
SANGEMINI minerale	TR	380 m	vetro	★	1020 □	21.9 ★	○	ricca di solfati
S. LUCIA minerale + CO_2	SS	228 m	vetro	★	1255 □	295 -	○	forte tenore di sodio, non adatta ad un uso quotidiano
S. PELLEGRINO minerale + CO_2	BG	358 m	PET	★	1065 □	41.1 □	○	forte tenore di solfati, non adatta ad un uso quotidiano
ULIVETO minerale	PI	12 m	PVC	★	1075 □	103.3 □	★	ricca di sodio, cloruri, solfati
Ricche di sali minerali (residuo superiore a 1500 mg/l)								
FERRARELLE minerale	CE	111 m	PET	□	1585 -	56.3 □	○	acqua dura, ricca di sodio
TETTUCCIO minerale	PT	29 m	vetro	★	6870 -	2257 -	○	forte tenore di sodio, non adatta ad un uso quotidiano se non secondo prescrizione medica

Chapter 30
Conditioned reflexes and obesity

«Remember that the best physician is Nature:
heals two-thirds of illnesses and does not speak ill of colleagues.»
Galen [Claudius Galen of Pergamum]

To work, an Orthomolecular Biohacking program must be simple, fun and efficacious in helping you achieve or regain your optimal fitness by shedding pounds of fat and perhaps gain muscle and new vital energy that you need to feel better! By feeling better you will appreciate yourself more, by improving your self-esteem you will be able to ignite the spark of constant improvement (Kaizen), the true pivot of this program and the engine of the constellation of your inner affective world! The organ that regulates self-esteem, according to Traditional Chinese Medicine (TCM), is the pancreas, which in turn modulates its function that synthesizes insulin, the hormone that regulates the amount of circulating sugar in the blood and consequently indirectly also the appetite.

Does the affective world of the obese explore different behavioral frequencies during the dream phase of sleep? Already during the waking phase, all negative emotions, such as anger and resentment, and positive emotions, such as joy and pleasure, can be mis-encoded by the obese and interpreted as an alarm message with the involvement of the neurovegetative system, which responds to the stress induced by these emotions with a rise in blood sugar at the expense of the cortico-adrenal system.

Such glycemic elevation is followed by an abrupt decrease in circulating sugars (hypoglycemia) that triggers a physiological immediate sensation

of hunger stress hypoglycemia with Pavlovian mode. The hunger stimulus is used to overcome glycemic fluctuations that put the individual survival. Eating to survive, to ultimately overcome the critical event using this atavistic reflex, often represented in an imperious and incoercible manner (hyperphagia). The conditioned reflex of compulsive hunger has clear and obvious scientific roots and is represented by the subject's response to the presentation of a conditioned stimulus, which is Pavlovian in nature.
The concept of conditioned reflex was introduced by Russian scientist Ivan Pavlov in the early twentieth century as part of behavioral studies. The conditioned reflex is a reaction produced in the captive animal by an external element that the animal becomes accustomed to associate with a specific stimulus (presented immediately, after or during the conditioning phase). The first agent therefore becomes the key stimulus, that which activates the conditioned reflex.

Ivan Petrovich Pavlov (1849-1936), Russian medical physiologist whose name is linked to the 1903 discovery of the conditioned reflex. He came to this discovery while, using dogs, conducting research on digestion: he already made such important contributions in this field that he earned the Nobel Prize in Medicine and Physiology in 1904. His classic experiment is well known: by associating the presentation of meat with a bell sound for a certain number of times, eventually the bell sound alone causes salivation (so-called mouth watering) in the dog, which it certainly did not produce before; thus the dog behaves this way because of a conditioned reflex artificially provoked in him. Pavlov's classical experiment aims to demonstrate the conditioned reflex, that is, with a stimulus one is able to cause the occurrence of a certain event (response). Organisms (animals and humans) learn to associate one stimulus with another. Central to classical conditioning are reflexes, i.e., unlearned responses, such as salivation, pupillary contraction, and eye closure.

The emotional and affective representation that the brain processes of the environmentally reactive need to introduce sugars after any kind of stress represents a Pavlovian compensatory mechanism. Pavlov prepared the conditioning phase: he fed the dog whenever the ringing of the bell occurred. After several repetitions, the bell stimulus was transformed into a conditioned stimulus capable of producing on its own a response, this time conditioned, of salivation.

→

The nocturnal raids on the refrigerator or pantry typical of the bulimic patient are easily explained. During night rest, for example, the onset of a nightmare puts the neurovegetative system on alert, which by releasing circulating stress hormones (adrenaline, etc.) unconsciously conditions the individual to seek food as an element atavistically related to the survival of the species.

Chapter 31

Deconditioning from bulimia

«... Then, more than sorrow, fasting could.» When he had said this, with his crooked eyes he resumed 'the miserable skull with his teeth,
Who were to the bone, as of a can, strong.»

Dante, Inferno, XXXIII, 75-78

Between food, emotions, and stress there is a deep, deep-rooted and inextricable link, which can sometimes result in the pathology of an eating disorder eating. This handbook OB can help you decondition yourself from compulsive (sudden and uncontrollable) hunger through the synergistic action of diet, supplements and exercise. Rebalancing these three parameters allows you to **«tranquilize»** the ventrolateral nucleus of the hypothalamus which acts as guardian of the neurovegetative life and the dense inner dialogue that a simple smell or flavor can arouse in the innermost areas of the brain.

Proust, too, in an episode of "In Search of Lost Time," refers to a close relationship between food and emotions through the concept of involuntary memory: the protagonist, dipping a madeleine in tea, feels an immense and inexpressible joy... In fact, the taste and flavor of tea and madeleines are able to make him relive the adolescent times he spent with his aunt in Combray. As if by magic, from a steaming cup of tea flow forth as if from a parallel universe places, people, colors and emotions that rational memory alone would not have been able to recall.

All this helps to understand how food intake holds a complex meaning that goes far beyond the purely physiological mechanism. Eating disorders place an emphasis on self-image, as a form organized in the way of seeing oneself projected and represented in the real world that begins to be structured from childhood through schemas that develop over time and based on experiential experience and that allow one to interpret actions, organize and plan memories and judgments.

To live and make a better person of oneself, each person has more or less creative potential. Three kinds of factors modulate its expression:

1. **Cognitive factors:** related to knowledge and mental faculties, stored information that facilitate creative thinking. All this information is processed throughout life through the education received, but also through the thread of personal experiences that are the real resource for facing challenges and difficult situations where change is needed;
2. **Conative factors:** related to individuals' personality traits, such as motivation, which confer "vis pugnandi," or the will to fight affintil things change;
3. **Environmental factors:** grouping the influence of family, parents, school, friends.

To be an executive you need to gain some knowledge in the area of your as yet unexpressed possibilities that will help you achieve the best results. First, focus well on divergent thinking, a mental process of producing many ideas from a single stimulus. The primary stimulus is definitely to want to live better and achieve mind-body balance. The more you are able to indulge in the flow of ideas in this manual, the more opportunities you will have to discover new and original ones in order to activate mental flexibility and the aptitude to find different solutions to a problem or otherwise consider it from another point of view. Ultimately, it is not a matter of multiplying ideational capacity, but of freeing oneself from the constraint of habitual thinking and regaining self-esteem by pursuing new goals, inherent in De Bono - Douglas creative lateral thinking.
The quality of cognitive flexibility is related to a neurotransmitter called «norepinephrine,» which has the ability to modulate the extent of neuronal networks recruited to perform a mental task. Extensive neural networks promote associations of ideas that allow for novel, and therefore creative, solutions to a problem such as excess body weight.
By associating ideas in an original way, you can deal with it better. The cre-

ative act that is needed whenever you face a new situation, such as the one you are facing now trying to change your life, requires the intervention of several brain structures. *The frontal cortex encourages the multiplication of ideas through divergent thinking, thanks to the associative neurons that promote exchange between the six layers of the cortex. The prefrontal cortex allows getting rid of an ineffective strategy, under the effect of the neuromodulator noradrenaline, secreted by the* ***locus coeruleus****.*
Finally, there is the corpus callosum, a bundle of fibers that connects the two hemispheres, enabling them to converse optimally by producing innovative ideas, an element that is indispensable for renewing old and poor strategies by replacing them with more effective and successful ones. From the primary need to acquire and preserve a positive self-image and the striving toward an «Ideal Self» discrepancies between the «Ideal Self» and the «Real Self» may emerge, based on past experiences. If this discrepancy is very strong, psychopathological processes, such as eating disorders, can be triggered. The self, from the somatic point of view, performs the function of a kind of identifying barcode, a credit card with which one puts oneself forward to the observation, evaluation and judgment of others. The evaluative severity of this judgment is somewhat proportional to body weight.

Today, the self-critical gaze can initiate extreme attempts to control body morphology through the performance of obsessive practices in the gym, cosmetic surgery, the use of drugs, and, first and foremost, food control such as orthorexia (see related chapter). People with eating disorders struggle every day to gain control over food that they are unable to acquire but are particularly trained and experienced in eliminating. A dualistic, perpetual and interminable conflict between two parts of the same being, where the "healthy" one allows itself to desire something, but at the very moment it gives in, the censorious, punitive, severe and primitive aspect of the other takes over.

The ultimate and innermost motive of extreme control is probably to pursue the complacent realization of an ideal, if subjective, self-image that does not necessarily correspond to the real good. What the boundary between normality and pathology might be is the challenge for the psyche that executes like a masterful director abrupt and sudden changes of scene, such as that of transforming an anorexic size 38 patient into a smug model of herself and her role.

The Western cultural system feeds the prodromes of a *dysmorphophobia*, of an anguished sense of not being beautiful, or of being disapproved of, already configurable as a preclinical situation, when the person cannot identify with pre constituted canons such as those proposed by fashion through sizes, a true discriminatory tool.

It bears a large share of responsibility for the media, having cheaply created flimsy, computer-corrected, computer-revised otherworldly myths of sculptural and excessively thin bodies: the myth of the eternal androgynous, while at the same time peppering us with false and tendentious advertisements promoting and advocating the purchase of fatty foods. All this creates chaos and confusion by increasing the gap between Ideal Body and Normal Body, generating anxiety that is reduced by controlling food. This is difficilly amendable, especially in the adolescent stage where one compares oneself with others and one's body image self-esteem is constantly changing due to the hormonal storm of puberty, thus making it fragile and undefined.

DECONDITIONING BY HACKING WITH AUTOGENIC TRAINING AND HYPNOSIS

Some thaumaturges of emotional dietetics, in order to reduce compulsion toward «dangerous» foods, make the intake of food associated with images that evoke disgust and revulsion in the patient; for example, being in front of a steaming plate of rigatoni with black olives and discovering, while one is eating, that the olives are actually cockroaches, which, once they reach the oral cavity, undergo the crushing of their chitinous skeleton against the dental cusps, pouring their semi-liquid, slimy, whitish internal substance into the mouth, flooding it. This methodology may well also be used just imaginatively, perhaps with the aid of concentration exercises such as autogenic training. The technique, which will turn the noses of many gastronomic purists, seems to ultimately yield good results and allows it to be personalized, as everyone feels revulsion for some things and for others does not and prefers some foods to others. The principle on which this method is based is to associate an extremely pleasant stimulus with one that is repulsive and unpleasant to the subject. It is, therefore, a true Pavlovian deconditioning technique that produces its results already in very few sessions, especially if they are carried out with a bi-weekly recall frequency.

Intervention on emotions is directly related to that of cognitive thinking analysis and consists, first of all, in knowing how to recognize and encode them in the right way.

It begins by learning to distinguish the main sensations of one's body-hunger, thirst, heat, cold, sleep, pain, etc. - by asking yourself precise and determined questions: What do I feel right now? What do I desire? Am I thirsty? Am I hungry?

All this involves considerable practice on the part of the patient who has never been trained to do so. Then we move on to the emotions: joy, pleasure, pain, anger, sadness, rejection, fear, etc., using the same process.

Cognitive intervention turns out to be the most important since it is the brain that processes and encodes internal and external information. (In this regard, it is assumed that our thinking, as early as the seventh year of life, is 75 percent structured, and based on direct experiences and received education, everyone forms a personal and subjective view of both the world and his or her inner self.)

The patient acquires a set of beliefs that he will tend to maintain more or less unchanged over time, since, through his behavior and his tendency to pay more attention to certain stimuli than to others, he will be inclined to generate self-confirmations, although often without being fully conscious and aware of them.

Chapter 32

Quantum Dots (Qds) Theranostic Technology

The future is here... grab it!

The author

The use of quantum technology to deliver drugs has the potential to increase the efficacy of many rare disease treatments. Semiconductor nanoparticles are a new type of treatment for life-threatening disorders.

The classical semiconductor quantum dots (QDs) are semiconductor particles that are able to emit fluorescence by excitation. The CQDs is mainly referred to photoluminescent carbon nanoparticles less than 10 nm, with surface modification or functionalization. Contrary to other carbon nanostructures, CQDs can be synthesized and functionalized fast and easily. The fluorescence origin of the CQDs is a controversial issue which depends on carbon source, experimental conditions, and functional groups. However, PL emissions originated from conjugated π-domains and surface defects have been proposed for the PL emission mechanisms of the CQDs. These nanostructures have been used as nontoxic alternatives to the classical heavy metals containing semiconductor QDs in some applications such as in-vivo and in-vitro bio-imaging, drug delivery, photosensors, chemiluminescence (CL), and etc.

The term «quantum dots:,QDs " refers to semiconductor nanoparticles. These quantum dots have a one-of-a-kind shape, size, fluorescence characteristics, and shape-dependent optoelectronic capacities. As a result, we believe that (QDs) has the potential to be destined as medication carriers, biosensors, etc.

Due to improvements in research, medicinal, and clinical domains, an in-depth examination of quantum dots is now possible.

Quantum dots are also classed as

- Carbon -based quantum dots,
- Grsphene-based quantum dots, and
- Cadmium-base quantum dots

Large variations in their main structure, leading to the discovery of more comparable and diversified quantum dots. Semiconductor quantum dots, or QDs, have also made tremendous progress in the field of fluorescence bioimaging research. After examining their in vitro and in vivo applications, we may currently use QDs as agents for gene transport, medication delivery, and enhancing the biocompatibility of other medications. Amazing breakthroughs and challenges in the field of quantum dots as biosensors for bioimaging, surface changes, quantum dots in the treatment of numerous diseases, and future features of quantum dots and their improvements in biomedical applications.

(*Quantum Dots as Theranostic Agents: Recent Advancements, Surface Modifications, and Future Applications Bhushan Phafat et al. Mini Rev Med Chem. 2023.*)

BASIC BIBLIOGRAPHY

* Carbon quantum dots with honeycomb structure: a novel synthesis approach utilizing cigarette smoke precursors. Setianto S, et al. Sci Rep. 2024. PMID: 38263381 Free PMC article.
* Tumor diagnosis using carbon-based quantum dots: Detection based on the hallmarks of cancer. Wang H, et al. Bioact Mater. 2023. PMID: 38034499 Free PMC article. Review.
* Comprehensive advances in the synthesis, fluorescence mechanism and multifunctional applications of red-emitting carbon nanomaterials. Mandal T, et al. Nanoscale Adv. 2023. PMID: 37881704 Free PMC article. Review.
* Carbon Dots-Types, Obtaining and Application in Biotechnology and Food Technology. Szczepankowska J, et al. Int J Mol Sci. 2023. PMID: 37834430 Free PMC article. Review.
* Luminescence of carbon quantum dots and their application in biochemistry. Bao H, et al. Heliyon. 2023. PMID: 37790961
* Luminescence of carbon quantum dots and their application in biochemistry.
* Bao H, et al. Heliyon. 2023. PMID: 37790961 Free PMC article. Review.
* Optical Properties of ScnYn (Y = N, P As) Nanoparticles.
* Michos FI, et al. Nanomaterials (Basel). 2023. PMID: 37764618 Free PMC article.

* Sensitive detection of cadmium ions based on a quantum-dot-mediated fluorescent visualization sensor.
* Ai Q, et al. RSC Adv. 2023. PMID: 37655354 Free PMC article.
* Disturbing cytoskeleton by engineered nanomaterials for enhanced cancer therapeutics.
* Xu X, et al. Bioact Mater. 2023. PMID: 37621771 Free PMC article. Review.
* Pure and doped carbon quantum dots as fluorescent probes for the detection of phenol compounds and antibiotics in aquariums.
* Mousa MA, et al. Sci Rep. 2023. PMID: 37553364 Free PMC article.

Chapter 33

Artificial intelligence: an OB approach

The real question is: when will we draft an AI bill of rights? What will it consist of? And who will be able to decide it?

Delfina Panfili, 2024

THE USE OF DIGITAL ASSISTANTS FOR ONE'S HOME

Home digital voice assistants in environments are «embodying the idea of a virtual butler who helps you 'get things done'» (Paay, et al., 2020, p. 30). To grasp the complexities of this project, it is critical to understand that the focus is on language processing software and machine learning algorithms that work by extracting data and information to perform specific tasks assigned by the user in the form of voice or text (Hoy , 2018). In addition, smart assistants are currently the flagship products in the smart home industry and one of the fastest and steadily growing technology projects in the past decade (Seymour et al., 2022). In fact, voice interaction with digital home assistants is considered one of the key developments in computing, reaching a point where it is predicted that by 2024, more than 57 million voice assistants will dominate European households.

Moreover, home voice assistants go beyond Internet of Things (IoT) devices as they are driven by machine learning and cloud computing that make users' experience with these digital assistants ubiquitous and smooth (De Conca, 2021). However, it is important to grasp the interconnectivity and deep relationship between IoT and smart technologies that include the ability to process, collect data, and respond to a given stimulus. Therefore, the focus is on the interdependence between devices of the user (IoT) that provides home assistants with personalized data and information that, in turn, will aim to completely resemble or mimic a form of cognition somewhat similar to human cognition. Therefore, the machine learning intelligence that powers home voice assistants is completely dependent on «the collection, processing and storage of personal data» (De Conca, 2021, p. 28). The exponential growth in the demand for personal voice assistants in the private sphere fuels a rather controversial discourse on whether the home can still be considered a place where behaviors are enacted with the certainty of not being observed or judged by others (Seymour et al., 2022). Moreover, the home implementation of such intelligent assistants may also raise social concerns that make the ethical aspect of technological design questionable.

HOME VOICE ASSISTANTS ADAPT TO CHANGING SOCIAL VALUES

The ubiquitous presence of the Artificial Internet of Things (AIoT), as well as its continued relevance in today's society, has sparked greater interest and desire from the manufacturing sector to adapt accordingly to the broader social and moral values that permeate society (Lin & Bergmann, 2016). However, research shows that although efforts have been made to achieve more inclusive and ethical technological design, there is still a long way to go.

The growing emphasis on diversity and inclusivity across gender, language, and culture has led smart assistant manufacturers to adapt to the changing social landscape (Cowls et al., 2019). Indeed, there has been a significant shift in the representation of the gendered voices of home assistants. That is, from a default female voice option that has fueled criticism for confirming stereotypes, gender biases, and social exclusion, has sprung ongoing efforts to enable voice assistants to represent and recognize multiple voices in terms of gender, language, and accents.

For example, the Google Assistant has successfully moved closer to a gender-neutral voice through a color naming system that implies countries will have a 50/50 chance of hearing orange or red Google voices (Statt, 2018). Voice assistants in the home are based on command and control systems, and a widely manifested value in the home environment is own control (De Conca, 2021). Specifically, the growth in the use of voice assistants at home has completely changed the way individuals make sense of and exercise control over their private sphere. Indeed, the research points out that technology as a whole is a key factor that has contributed to this radical change in the perception of privacy. That is, in the case of values such as control and privacy, the focus is on how both technology and society together adapt, reinvent and constitute social reality. In particular, home environments and privacy have been severely eroded such that the home is no longer seen as a place where one's personality, habits, and identity characteristics can manifest freely with the knowledge that one has control over the environment. In contrast, voice assistants have the ability to reduce the extent to which inhabitants feel they have control over particular home environments, caused by the continuous collection of data and processing of personal information. Therefore, control over private spheres of life is now seen as a double-edged sword wielded by both the voice assistant and its users (Statt, 2018).

Despite these changing perceptions about what control entails in the context of voice assistants, various technology companies have introduced ethical guidelines and procedures that ensure levels of accountability and consensus (De Conca, 2021). For example, the Google Assistant is working on a set of artificial intelligence principles that demonstrate their commitment to establishing responsible, transparent, and ethical technology design (Statt, 2018). In addition, accessibility is another social value that is gaining great relevance as it plays an important role in assessing the extent to which artificial intelligence designs are ethically sound in terms of their ability to function and serve a global and diverse user group (Park et al., 2022). Therefore, it implies that voice assistant manufacturers will be able to develop ways that enable people with differences in access and use, such as people with disabilities, to make use of intelligent assistants. In fact, research shows that designers of voice assistants are implementing building blocks in technology design that make it accessible to people with disabilities. For example, Amazon's Alexa is now considered a functional tool for users with visual impairments as it can be used with screen readers and voice over systems (Barry, 2021).

Overall, the continuous evolution of voice assistants can be seen both as a response to changing social values, but also as a constitutive element of this change (Guess, 2017). On the one hand, voice assistants adapt and attempt to reflect social values. On the other hand, the design of the technology inevitably alters and reinvents aspects of the social world. Therefore, despite these positive developments, contemporary discourses concerning the broader ethical sphere need to be grasped in order to imagine a more inclusive and responsible design of voice assistants.

The brain is like a large orchestra and today, with new technologies, we are able to listen to it better, and understand the "variations" on the theme: these are the key themes of Mnesys, a project dedicated to the in-depth study of neuronal plasticity and its connectivity. Create an avatar of the brain, a digital double that allows us to predict the progression of the disease in each patient or how he or she will react to treatment.

A challenge that starts from the awareness that «the brain is plastic, and in a constant state of learning (even if damaged) and can continuously learn some-

thing new and adapt to the environment, thus also managing to compensate for the initial damage of diseases such as Parkinson's or multiple sclerosis.
Plasticity always manifests itself as a structural or functional modification of the connections between neurons: brain functions are not the result of the activation of a single neuron nor of a group localized in a specific area. The brain functions through neural networks organized on different scales of complexity: molecular and cell membrane processes determine the activity of neurons, which influence that of neuronal microcircuits, which then associate in larger networks. By analyzing this complexity, Mnesys researchers managed to obtain multiscale digital representations of neurons, microcircuits, neural networks and the entire brain, starting from magnetic resonance imaging that allow functional areas to be mapped on a digital brain atlas: digital avatars can replicate the behavior of the brain and generate, for example, brain waves very similar to those of an electroencephalogram, allowing the brain functions that emerge in the case of neurological diseases to be studied in detail.
The next step is the digital twins of the brains of individual patients by processing the available data through mathematical algorithms: this will allow us to simulate functional states and neural parameters that are not detectable with clinical and diagnostic evaluations and will be able to help improve diagnoses, predict the evolution of the disease to define more appropriate and personalized treatments.

PRIVACY THREATS

In assessing the extent to which smart assistants are designed to be socially valuable tools, a key factor that has attracted much criticism is privacy (Cowls et al., 2019). Exploratory research outlines how user skepticism stems from misunderstandings about how personal data collection processes work. Specifically, most users do not trust the manufacturers and prices of the devices available to them. For example, studies have shown that information made accessible to users about recording processes such as VA microphone muting makes the belief that the digital tool constantly listens to its users even more credible (Seymour et al., 2022). In addition, qualitative research also investigates how privacy issues arise due to the inability of voice assistants to distinguish different voices. Specifically, the ability of VAs to automatically purchase items if asked to do so is a factor of concern with regard to safety status (Cowls et al., 2019). In fact, empirical research shows that failure to recognize differences between voice profiles is one of the main reasons associated with levels of usage restraint within multi-dwelling household spheres (Seymour et al., 2022). Lack of user trust regarding hidden features of voice assistants, as well as security concerns, are constituents of a violation of human dignity, a key aspect to consider when assessing the extent to which digital tools are responsibly designed.

CONCLUSIONS

Overall, this narrative opens up the debate on whether it is possible to imagine inclusive and ethical design of voice assistants households, making them accessible to a diverse and global user group. With an optimistic approach, designers of digital AI tools should focus on providing users with a more transparent procedure on how VA processes and stores personal data. Recognizing that the most recurring sentiment evoked in VA users is that of «not knowing enough» about digital technology, it is certain that greater levels of transparency between VA offerings and users would increase their trust, knowledge, and trustworthiness. (Pradhan, 2019, p.15). Moreover, to regain some of the control that individuals have lost, designers could potentially constitute a personalized experience with voice assistants. Specifically, reflecting the needs and preferences of a specific group of users could make them feel a greater level of dominance and control over their digital tool. However, personalizing the experience of individuals could involve extracting even more personal data to enable the technology to function according to user preferences.

Therefore, transparency and personalization are elements that would reinvent home voice assistants and could potentially improve attitudes toward issues such as data surveillance, lack of control, and privacy violations. Taking a pessimistic approach and in line with Bourdieu's theory, «the reproduction of inequalities is a reflection of socially entrenched sets of practices accessible only to people with distinctive socioeconomic resources» (Park et al., 2022, p. 2). Therefore, it is clear that to solve the problems related to inequalities in access, and to envision an ethical technological project, a change needs to be implemented among the fundamental layers of society such as culture, economics, and politics. Therefore, on a global scale, it seems quite difficult to create an ethical artificial intelligence project, as ethics is deeply interconnected with society and the values on which it is based.

Bibliographic references

Barry, W. (n.d.). How alexa benefits individuals who are blind or visually impaired. Bridging apps alt. Retrieved March 28, 2023, from.

https://bridgingapps.org/how-alexa-benefits-individuals-who-are-blind- or-visually-impaired

Cowls, J., King, T., Taddeo, M., & Floridi, L. (2019). Designing AI for social good: Seven essential factors. SSRN Electronic Journal. https://doi.org/10.2139/ssrn.3388669

De Conca, S. (2021). The enchanted house: An analysis of the interaction of intelligent personal home assistants (IPHAs) with the private sphere and its legal protection.

Guess, A. R. (2017, May 21). Virtual Digital assistants to overtake World Population by 2021. DATAVERSITY. Retrieved March 17, 2023, from https://www.dataversity.net/virtual-digital-assistants-overtake-world- population-2021/.

Hagerty, A., & Rubinov, I. (2019). Global Ai Ethics: A Review of the Social Impacts and Ethical Implications of Artificial Intelligence (dissertation). Cornell University. https://arxiv.org/pdf/1907.07892.pdf

Hoy, M. B. (2018). Alexa, Siri, Cortana, and more: An introduction to voice assistants. Medical Reference Services Quarterly, 37(1), 81-88. https://doi.org/10.1080/02763869.2018.1404391

Lin, H., & Bergmann, N. (2016). IOTprivacyandsecuritychallengesfor Smart Home Environments. Information, 7(3), 44. https://doi.org/10.3390/info7030044.
Paay, J., Kjeldskov, J., Hansen, K. M., Jørgensen, T., & Overgaard, K. L. (2020). Digital Ethnography of home use of digital personal assistants. Behaviour & Information Technology, 41(4), 740-758. https://doi.org/10.1080/0144929x.2020.1834620

Park, Y. J., Lee, H., Jones-Jang, S. M., & Oh, Y. W. (2022). Digital assistants: Inequalities and social context of access, use, and Perceptual Understanding. Poetics, 93, 101689. https://doi.org/10.1016/j.poetic.2022.101689.

Pradhan, A. (2018). Exploring the Accessibility of Home-Based, Voice- controlled Intelligent Personal Assistants (Order No. 10793196). Available from ProQuest

Dissertations & Theses Global; ProQuest Dissertations & Theses Global. (2078904629). https://www.proquest.com/dissertations-theses/exploring-accessibility- home-based-voice/doc view/2078904629/se-2

Pridmore, J., Zimmer, M., Vitak, J., Mols, A., Trottier, D., Kumar, P. C., & Liao, Y. (2019). Intelligent personal assistants and the intercultural negotiations of Dataveillance in platformed households. Surveillance & Society, 17(1/2), 125-131. https://doi.org/10.24908/ss.v17i1/2.12936

Seymour, W., & Van Kleek, M. (2021). Exploring interactions between trust, anthropomorphism, and relationship development in voice assistants. Proceedings of the ACM on Human-Computer Interaction, 5(CSCW2), 1-.
16. https://doi.org/10.1145/3479515

Seymour, W., Cote, M., & Such, J. (2022). Can you meaningfully consent in eight seconds? identifying ethical issues with verbal consent for voice assistants. 4th Conference on Conversational User Interfaces. https://doi.org/10.1145/3543829.3544521

Statt, N. (2018, July 10). Google now refers to its different assistant voices using colors. The Verge. Retrieved March 28, 2023, from https://www.theverge.com/2018/7/10/17556692/google-assistant- voices-color-coding-scheme -ai

Szczuka, J. M., Strathmann, C., Szymczyk, N., Mavrina, L., & Krämer, N. C. (2022). How do children acquire knowledge about voice assistants? A longitudinal field study on children's knowledge about how voice assistants store and Process Data. International Journal of Child-Computer Interaction, 33, 100460. https://doi.org/10.1016/j.ijcci.2022.100460.
Xu, S., & Li, W. (2022). A tool or a social being? A Dynamic Longitudinal Investigation of functional use and relational use of AI Voice assistants. New Media & Society, 146144482211081. https://doi.org/10.1177/14614448221108112.

Delfina Panfili

Doctor of Digital Communication King's College University London UK

https://www.linkedin.com/in/delfina-panfili-a9939a244/ panfilidelfina@gmail.com

Chapter 34
The energy of light

«We can forgive a child when he is afraid of the dark.
The real tragedy of life is when a man is afraid of the light.»

Plato

Light is as indispensable a source of energy to our bodies as the water we drink and the air we breathe. Sunlight produces enormous effects on our psycho-emotional state, on dopaminergic hormonal cascades from which the urge to do and to be springs. Enormous are the repercussions on every aspect of human physiology, beauty and potential longevity. However, there are currents that claim that the sun can be a cause of neoplasms, aging early, damage to skin and eyesight.

To settle these paradoxical norms, it is useful to quote the summary of the courageous indictment of Franco Berlin, former Director of the Department of Biomedical Sciences at the National Cancer Institute in Milan.

«Let's put it this way, if we don't get sick the GDP increases, and if there is growth the spread decreases.

Health care is the largest national industry. As Professor Monti saw fit to remind us, there is no direct economic interest in prevention. What word could be used to define it? It is a committee of ignorance and stupidity and interests...».

LIGHT, A PRECIOUS DRUG

Sunlight is the most powerful natural medicine that Mother Nature has freely granted to man.

It is no coincidence that the main religious cults have always turned to solar deities beginning with the Egyptians, the pre-Christian Mithraic cults, Toltec, Hindu, Tibetan, Islamic, and Jewish... Why this belated and incomprehensible demonization of life itself that has its primal roots in the sun and stars?

Think of the skin as a wonderful apparatus covered with solar panels, capable of directly or indirectly converting some chemically simple substances such as cholesterol into life-critical substances such as vitamin D, such as growth hormone and testosterone, the latter hormone being crucial for the vitality, sexuality, and productivity of both men and women. The evolutionary phylogeny of the species is brought about through the effect of light, and all scripture begins with the fateful phrase «...and it was light»!

> Just think that the ultraviolet rays naturally present in the total sunlight spectrum (even in winter when the sky is apparently cloudy) are able to break the double ring of cholesterol and convert it into vitamin D3, male and female hormones, serotonin (hormone that regulates sugar metabolism). Serotonin is that precious molecule that, when present, makes us see the glass half full; when deficient, it makes us see it half empty.

During winter it is well known that blood cholesterol levels increase due to decreased sun exposure, often causing increases in fat mass and increased ghrelin which in turn reduces insulin efficiency.
Over the past four decades there has been a progressive lower exposure of humans to ultraviolet light resulting in a lowering of the average testosterone value scientifically considered a «normal fluctuation»; for a male adult it is hard to believe how a 60 percent drop in the concentration of a hormone such as testosterone can be considered «normal» in four decades.
Now add to this the lowered serotonin concentration (SAD syndrome: Seasonal Affective Disorder).
While darkness saddens, the sun awakens. After the onset of spring, the sun awakens nature's hibernation with broad-spectrum light from the sun by stimulating oestrus, the mating of all beings that respond to the metabolic-hormonal stimulus that light exerts on each organism. The ultraviolet light contained in the total sunlight spectrum activates circadian biorhythms (light-dark effect) by modulating the action of the epiphyseal gland (the one that goes haywire when we take an intercontinental flight and experience jet lag).
The biological clocks that regulate meridian function in Chinese culture are activated by the synthesis of vitamin D, which is capable of fixating calcium in bones but also enhancing emotional states by improving serotonin metabolism in the gut, for regulation of metabolism, and prevention of cancer and cardiovascular issues.

Think that even according to some, inhibiting this light could greatly increase the wealth for the disease industry... **«honni soit qui mal y pense»** «onì suà ki mal i pãs» (fr. ant. **«be shamed he who thinks ill»**). This famous motto of the English Order of the Garter was instituted, according to a legendary tradition, by King Edward III of England in honor of his own mistress, the Countess of Salisbury, to whom a garter had fallen during a ball; the king rushed to pick it up and reprimanded with such words the courtiers who smiled at the episode.

I agree with Prof. Fabio Marchesi when he states that there is no scientifically proven evidence that sunlight and ultraviolet rays can be harmful to human beings. This would be one of the most colossal lies ever perpetrated and disseminated globally in the history of human civilization. In fact, sunlight and ultraviolet light can really only do harm to the revenues of unscrupulous multinational corporations in chemistry, pharmacology, such as those marketing drugs for cholesterol reduction, impotence, depression, which benefit enormously from the spread of hypothetical problems related to insufficient exposure to sunlight.

One of the most "authoritative" studies ever cited aimed at penalizing and reducing ultraviolet entitled "Action Spectrum for Retinal Injury from Ultraviolet Radiation in the Aphakic Monkey "was conducted in 1981 at the Medical College of Virginia. These scientists, in order to succeed in proving that ultraviolet actually damaged the retina, had to shine a Xenon lamp with high dosages of ultraviolet equal to 2500 W for a time period of 100 and 1000 seconds (more than 16 minutes) into three open monkey eyes from the laboratory from which the lens had first been surgically removed; the results of this disgraceful experimentation were used to scientifically prove that ultraviolet rays damage the retina, to prevent people, at least those who wear glasses, from receiving ultraviolet in their eyes, making people believe that it is for their own good. This experimentation has led to banning and making illegal any prescription sunglasses without ultraviolet filters, despite the fact that other research has shown the importance of the presence of ultraviolet in the light reaching the eyes in maintaining visual efficiency, the vitality of the cones and rods as well as regulating all hormonal and metabolic functions.

What a pity that many ophthalmic physicians and dermatologists limit themselves to reading only the headlines and results of the experiments that are brought to their attention, without taking an interest in how and with what intent they may have been conducted; by searching one can also find research that has shown, for example, that if the lens is not surgically removed, the retina of monkey eyes does not suffer injury even when exposed to natural dosage of ultraviolet.

Science teaches all of us the power of ideas and imagination, but also that we must learn to learn every day.
There is, however, alas, also a commoditized partisan science in the service of multinational pharmaceutical corporations that have become so wealthy and powerful that they are able to place their pawn men in neuralgic and strategic positions in the academic and popularization system, so as to condition any mass media to publish the results of certain research rather than others.
The ultimate goal of science is the understanding and modeling of nature in order to be able to predict the development of one or more phenomena. Prediction certainly does not mean preemptively imposing an asset of results. Every scientific theory develops a model that allows the mathematical or, more generally, rational representation of the phenomenon in order to be able to make predictions.
With the advent of Artificial Intelligence already foreshadowed by Pauling during a memorable dinner with Prof. Abram Hoffer, technological innovation would continuously open up unprecedented scenarios. It does, in fact, break existing balances in line with the evolving reality. It is this nature of technology that constrains us to be creative, to shift the axis of our thinking.
Prof. Pauling asserted that what seemed clear to us in linear logic is suddenly no longer so. Indeed, in an increasingly complex world, the evolution and interrelatedness of challenges place us at the door of new beginnings and tell us, in fact, that the paradigms we used to use in the world behind us no longer apply.
A science that is static, predictable and influenceable by government funding and patronage for public fundraising no longer qualifies as such.

The conditioning of beliefs and the collective action of the conditioned masses cannot be superimposed on a true model of free, independent and creative science.

In conclusion, according to Marchesi, health care is not about health, but about maximizing the economic exploitation of disease.
The results of meager research aimed at demonstrating the danger of ultraviolet rays naturally present in sunlight have been strangely disseminated with great emphasis throughout the world through pseudo-scientific channels, to the point of convincing everyone to banish them from their existence, avoid them and protect themselves from them despite a multitude of other far more reliable and more scientifically impactful, but undisclosed, studies demonstrating instead exactly the opposite.
The end result of this sordid alchemy is a population that is all the more weak, unhappy, overweight and consuming greater amounts of drugs.
We live in environments lit by artificial light that prefers vibrational frequencies of orange, which certainly have an illuminating effect but do not provide the full spectrum of sunlight required for perfect mammalian biofunctionality.

ENVIRONMENT AND LIGHTING
Ambient lighting prefers frequencies that do not produce ultraviolet light. Since little UV passes through glass windows, and outdoors it is customary to wear goggles that block it, and when we expose ourselves to the sun we have been educated to put on creams with chemical filters that prevent the skin from reaping its beneficial effects well... You draw your own conclusions.
I often recommend the use in home environments the use of lamps such as OSRAM's ultra-life Lux with high light saturation around 30,000 lux to ensure the minimum light requirement of the total solar spectrum to nourish and ensure the essential biochemical functions of the human body. In an environment where Lux saturation below is 2500 lux, for example, vitamin D3 biosynthesis is slowed and frankly inhibited. When you eat breakfast, don't forget to turn on the broad-spectrum solar light to recharge your batteries. Orthomolecular Biohacking is the art of changing the environment around and within us to have full control of our bodies and brains.
Various research shows that light plays a key role in sending messages to the mitochondria. In fact, light indicates what to do and when. Light is not

only a nutrient, since we have been using it in medicine for a hundred years, but it may even be identifiable as a drug.

In women in particular, after the brain, heart and ovaries, the eyes represent the highest concentration of mitochondria, which is why the eyes are extremely sensitive to anything that interferes with their energy production.
When the energy supply to the mitochondria in the eyes is inadequate, one can suffer from mental clouding, headaches, and even lose the ability to identify shades of gray.
The eyes acquire an enormous amount of information, and the brain needs a lot of energy to process and make sense of it; therefore, if the eyes are forced to function in an environment with a light and unnatural spectrum they are subjected to stress, and then energy production slows down, increasing the creation of free radicals, and they too can be damaged. As a result, the brain has more difficulty processing the light information absorbed by the eyes, and this is likely to impair its performance, since the mitochondria communicate with each other, and any stress to which they are subjected adversely affects the brain, heart and other parts of the body. This is precisely why it is necessary to identify the best way to illuminate one's environment so as to improve the function of the mitochondria.

HARMFUL LIGHT AS A HARMFUL FOOD

It is said that food stimulates appetite and that appetite comes with eating, but actually it comes with fasting. By changing natural light sources today we are compromising our biology, and the mitochondria are suffering because it is not the right brightness in which they evolved. As early as 1961 John Ott discovered the dangers of certain light frequencies, and best-selling author Dr. Teresa Wiley also talks in her books about the disturbances that bad lighting can create to health.

> In our quest for maximum energy savings, we have created artificial lights with a mixture of light frequencies that our bodies do not recognize; we have eliminated infrared light, which has a wavelength just above the red limit of the visible spectrum, that is, the electromagnetic spectrum of light visible to the human eye. Ultraviolet light, therefore, cannot be seen but is perceived in the form of heat: it is the invisible part of the sunlight spectrum and is essential for living things and also, of course, for our mitochondria.

Today, we prevent ultraviolet A and B rays from reaching our eyes with windshields, glasses and sunglasses and our skin with protective creams. This also affects the whole body, because the eyes are not the only ones that absorb light; the skin also absorbs light in its cells and mitochondria. There are good reasons for filtering out some UVA and UVB rays, because overexposure of the skin causes sunburn, while overexposure of the eyes can lead to vision damage.It is thought that excessive use of ultraviolet light is harmful and that is why we tend to eliminate it altogether, but this is not in our best interest, because our body needs a certain amount of this light to function better; in fact, ultraviolet rays are essential to activate vitamin D in the body and to help circadian rhythms, those physiological processes that regulate sleep-wake rhythms. Great strides have been made to save on electricity with high-efficiency devices, but these innovations send the mitochondria into meltdown, as mentioned above. This is bad light and can be comparable to food that is not good for us.

Exposure in the evening to artificial light has a negative impact on the circadian rhythm, whereas, on the other hand, when the body is in daylight it produces serotonin, the "good mood" neurotransmitter, and converts it into melatonin, a sleep-promoting hormone.

Many people think they sleep properly because they sleep 8 hours, but when they wake up they have no energy. This because the quality of sleep is more important than the quantity. Exposing oneself to artificial light when darkness has fallen slows down the production of melatonin, preventing quality sleep and also causing one to gain weight. Lack of sleep and weight gain both result in mitochondrial inefficiency.

RED LIGHT

«The chromatic alteration that the sun takes in its daily cycle has existed since before mammals populated the planet; therefore, we have evolved following this rhythm, our circadian rhythm.»

A.P.

The bacteria that make up our mitochondria today floated in the ocean where they were bathed in sunlight during the day, and they function by following this same circadian rhythm, because they are what regulate us. During the day, when eating a lot, they stay awake to eat and produce energy while at night they sleep to recharge.

Mitochondria are made to receive red light all day long with less blue light at the beginning and end of the day. When we spend time outdoors, our eyes and the mitochondria there are exposed to light that contains the full spectrum of light. Unfortunately, we spend little time outside today absorbing sunlight, and our mitochondria suffer. When we are indoors we receive blue light but no red or infrared light; therefore, the mitochondria become confused and do not work in the most high-performance way. Dr. Gerald Pollack, professor of Bioengineering at the University of Washington, has found that infrared light transforms the water in our bodies and plants on a biological level because it promotes mitochondrial function. Water should be abundant in cells, but the toxins we ingest with food and absorb from the environment as well as bad light alter their structure, causing inflammation and impairing energy production. Our body is made up of 70% water, and if light changes this water it also has the power to change us. For all these reasons, exposing ourselves to natural light is crucial for the brain to function well, and we should be aware that many new technologies can help us replicate the natural cycle: using a strip of red LED lights can counterbalance the excess blue frequencies that characterize technological devices, or another way to increase exposure to healthy light is to take an ultra-red sauna.

- They reduce the risk of retinal degeneration and reduced vision: in the eyes, retinal cells do not divide and regenerate without a small amount of ultraviolet light.
- They are effective in treating psoriasis: the National Psoriasis Foundation reports that 80 percent of psoriasis sufferers improve when exposed to UV light.
- They are effective in treating a number of other conditions, including asthma, respiratory problems, and tuberculosis.
- They reduce the risk of retinal degeneration and reduced vision: in the eyes, retinal cells do not divide and regenerate without a small amount of ultraviolet light.
- They are effective in treating psoriasis: the National Psoriasis Foundation reports that 80 percent of psoriasis sufferers improve when exposed to UV light.

- They are effective in treating a number of other conditions, including asthma, respiratory problems, and tuberculosis.

- They improve sex hormone levels (testosterone and estrogen) due to UV-8.
- They improve the effectiveness of the immune system.
- They reduce the risk of cardiovascular disease.
- They improve fitness, strength, and physical performance.

EFFECTS OF PROPER REGULAR EXPOSURE TO ULTRAVIOLET RAYS

They activate vitamin D synthesis, for proper absorption of calcium, minerals and amino acids, activating metabolism and stabilizing the ortho and parasympathetic neurovegetative symptoms.

- They reduce blood pressure (BP) by improving the efficiency of the heart muscle.
- Exposure to ultraviolet light was shown to reduce BP from the first treatment, and these effects persisted for another 56 days. In addition, in 90% of the subjects tested, cardiac efficiency increased by 39%.
- It improves electrocardiographic (ECG) tracing and blood values, especially in subjects with atherosclerosis.
- They reduce cholesterol, and 97% of the subjects studied lowered circulating cholesterol levels by 13% two hours after the first exposure, 86% maintaining the lowest level until twenty-four hours after exposure.
- They stimulate metabolism and contribute to weight reduction through thyroid stimulation of the endocrine system.

Chapter 35
OB of light: the red light life...

«The red sole of my shoes is like a handkerchief that an elegant woman drops if she has seen a man who attracts her.»

Christian Louboutin

Life on earth originated from physical carbonaceous skeleton elements called amino acids: the so-called building blocks of proteins (see *Orthomolecular Medicine: a human-friendly therapy* - Ed. New Techniques).
The amino acids that appear most frequently in the protein structures of living organisms are called ordinary or proteinogenic amino acids. Although more than 500 types of amino acids are known in nature, there are 20 ordinary L-amino acids.
On such mosaic tiles of life your livelihood depends. The very roots of human beings consist of biological processes inherited from your animal ancestors in turn from the plant world that had taken them from the mineral world. These three types of evolution-inorganic, biological and psychosocial, while boasting countless aspects in common, operate on distinct and transcendent principles. Organic chemistry will not be able to illustrate the life processes of cells, even though each cellular process is the consequence of chemical interactions. Similar reasoning applies to zoology, which, while considering the countless parallels between Homo Erectus and the great anthropomorphic great apes, will not be able to assess human merits in detail. Arrhenius in his (1898) paper titled «Cosmic Influences on Physiological Phenomena» claimed the existence of lunar influence on births, deaths, seizures and menstrual flow in women. Newton's gravitational interaction between the moon and sun on the water mass of the seas induces a periodic, regular and constant oscillation that provides over the course of the lunar day (duration of 24 hours and 50 minutes)

two rises and two falls. It is permissible to consider tides as extended waves with a period of 12 hours and 25 minutes, or 44,676 seconds.
Due to the thermal convection of huge air masses, tidal dynamics involves large variations in atmospheric pressure. The rhythm of the human respiratory rate is the harmonic of the tidal wave being in clear resonance with it, as can be inferred from the fact that the period of respiratory acts is 13,000 times smaller than that of the tides:

44,676 / 13,000 = 3.43 seconds

Similarly, the dynamics of blood fluids in the human body seem to resonate with the syzygial rhythm of the tides. In fact, it turns out that as a result of the displacement of huge masses and volumes of water, tidal currents develop in the seas, the forward speed of which would be about 0.5 m/sec corresponding to the speed of blood flow within arterial and venous vessels (10 cm/sec in veins and 20-40 cm/sec in arteries).
These considerations suggest that heart rate and respiratory rate would be periodic phenomena proportional to the rate of tidal sigicial wave of advancement.

OB: THE WOMAN, THE WATER AND THE MOON

Since the female organism is richer in water than males, it will respond like the oceans more sensitively to the changes in gravitational attraction found during the lunar synodic month, creating the cyclical pattern of menstrual flow. It is no coincidence, then, that the human menstrual cycle is the same length as the lunar menstrual cycle, or about 29 1/2 days.
The duration of gestation corresponds to 9 lunar months, or 265.8 days, according to a study performed in 1959 by Menaker on a sample of 250,000 births.
Even the process of reproduction would be marked by astronomical rhythms external to the intrinsic biology of the human cell.
The changing position of the moon relative to the sun is also responsible for changes in the environment and behavior that have been known for centuries.
The irregularity of cycles in many cases may be correlated with exposure to light during the night, that is, with an incorrect synchronization of the circadian melatonin secretory rhythm with the full moon phase.

Women with dysmenorrhea by simply turning on low lux red lights during the night of the 14th-15th-16th day can regularize their flow without resorting to medication.

Simple coincidences, or obvious observation that the physiological functions of the human organism resonate with the vital, pulsating activity of the Earth understood as a living organism, endowed with energy flowing through it along preferential lines, analogous to the acupuncture meridians of the human body.

Advancing the theory of cosmozoa (Panspermia, ed.) Arrhenius hypothesized the transmission of life from one planet to another through living va-grant microorganisms from star to star of incredible endurance, capable of tolerating the enormous temperatures emitted by celestial bodies. Red light also helps improve mood and feel-good hormones such as sero-tonin, endorphins, and acetylcholine, as well as reduce inflammation, im-prove circulation, and increase stem sparing and collagen production for healthy skin and a glowing complexion.

Commonly referred to as RLT (Red Light Therapy), photobiomodulation was accidentally discovered by Endre Mester in 1967 at Semmelweis Med-ical University in Budapest, Hungary; he noticed that laser light helped stimulate hair regrowth and wound repair in rats.

Red light was then studied for its potential therapeutic application during space travel by NASA and ESA. The researchers hoped it could help treat muscle atrophy, slow wound healing and bone density problems caused by prolonged weightlessness in space.

When photons (light particles) are placed near the skin, they penetrate the tissue and activate chromophores (a part of a molecule that gives it color), triggering changes in the cells, according to the American Society for Laser Medicine & Surgery.

In addition, RLT (red light therapy) also impacts by charging electrons the mitochondria (the powerhouse of cells), generating ATP (energy) to promote healing, as observed by the PBM Foundation.

DERMATOLOGICAL USE OF RLT

Red light therapy is promoted as a treatment for some common skin conditions, including:

- It improves wound healing.
- Reduce stretch marks
- Reduce wrinkles, fine lines and age spots.
- It improves the structure of the face.

- Improves psoriasis, rosacea and eczema.
- Improves scars.
- Improves sun-damaged skin.
- Improving hair growth in people with androgenetic alopecia.
- Improves acne.

Science shows that red lenses with "junk light" blocking technology are the most effective option for inducing faster and deeper sleep.
Yellow and orange increase contrast and look great on snow. Green reduces glare. Brown tones block blue light and increase contrast with grass and sky. Reddish hues can be calming and suitable for long car rides.
Red lenses are the most effective in promoting better sleep at night. Consider using red lenses to block the maximum amount of blue, green and violet light during the night that would interfere with non-Rem sleep. Better sleep to feel better in the aftermath!

Chapter 36

The music that heals (Healing Music)

If music is love nourishment of love, keep playing so that my heart falls ill and dies, oh, spirit of love, how alive and fresh you are! So multiform love presents itself, to be, he alone, the triumph of fantasy.

Duke Oisino, The Twelfth Night, or what you will
(William Shakespeare 1564-1616)

It all started not with light, but with a sound explosion: all of us, but also the oceans, the trees, Jupiters, the comets are immersed in a universe of sounds and radiation.
Acoustics, that strange science with uncertain boundaries that often relegate it to an ancillary and secrated role, do not always allow it to occupy the place that does not always make it count on the podium of the exact sciences, outlines a path that spreads in space and at the same time creates its own environment. Since the air once invaded by the acoustic vibrations that propagate in it, whether those of a clapping of hands or a piano sonata, they induce quantum significant changes of the primordial ether making it different from what it was before... remember the quantum aphorism: "If a butterfly flaps wings in Hong Kong In New York the air is moved...". What would it be like to rediscover this invisible but real sound ocean that has always resonated within each of us?
What else is possible?
Why not sing this wonderful symphony in which we are immersed from birth?
We have been immersed in music for a long time before our birth and there is a sound perception during intrauterine life.
Every acoustic phenomenon is nothing more than an echo of the primordial sound, of that immense explosion from which everything, just everything began, including even the magnificent unforgettable Mozart symphonies that our ears are able to hear.

With over 100 billion neurons constantly using Popp's ultra-weak biophotonic mitochondrial modulation to communicate with each other, the brain has become a large information sorting hub like New York's Grand Central Station.
Imagine for a moment that you are right in this very crowded underground bus station and obviously remarkable, clearly if everyone is chatting loudly at the same time, it can be difficult to focus on the coo we need to do.
Precisely in this context that we can use the MUSICAL OB
(Musical biohacking, nda) . Brain activity can be measured according to a wave pattern and determines our state of alertness, sopor, relaxation, stress.

There are numerous frequencies that can affect brain waves including the activity that takes place, the restorative rest, what you have just eaten or drunk.

One of the most reliable and effective ways to modify brain waves and precisely through the administration of a wave.

One of the most reliable ways to modify brain waves is through a coherent sound wave and music.

Audio drag, a form of musical biohacking, uses binaural beats and tones to synchronise with brain waves and induce a meditative and relaxed state (Alpha/ Theta Waves Driving Music)

As a kind of tailor-made tailored dress you can access programs developed specifically for the brain and the activities you want to perform.

And I also know to everyone how much listening to a good piece of music can modulate one's mood in a positive and sometimes therapeutic sense.

So why not create your own favourite playlist and listen to it while you train, prepare breakfast or go to work?

MOZART EFFECT AND DOPAMINE

The theory of the Mozart effect on the brain is based on the fact that listening to music (and, in particular, relaxing music) allows us to increase our level of **dopamine: the "neutransmitter of happiness"**, coming into action, would in fact improve our cognitive performance, making us more attentive and free to store new information. Do you raise your hand who has never listened to music to stimulate concentration, perhaps in the middle of a pre-exam study session? Hence another epithet of classical music: it is also called cognitive music, so called because it stimulates cognitive functions and facilitates learning abilities. The dopamine in the body and the consequent state of happiness and satisfaction have made sure to define classical music also as 'an antidepressant music': able to calm states of anxiety and fear, it is in fact to influence our emotional state and therefore raise our mood.

A decade after Rauscher and Shaw's theory, Professor John Jenkins of the University of London published an article entitled "The Mozart Effect" in the journal of the Royal Society of Medicine, according to which he demonstrated the positive effects of music on the treatment of several diseases. According to a development of this theory of the Mozart effect, **Mozart's sonata K448 would even have a beneficial effect on epilepsy**, as it would lead to a reduction in the frequency of the most acute seizures. If this theory has long been opposed by the majority of members of the international medical community, it can also be said that it has been proven that music therapy has, in general, a strong impact on children and behavioural psychology. Music therapy (that is, the use of music and the use of musical instruments) has a strong impact on communication, motor skills, expression, sociability and learning from an early age.

Chapter 37

Genetics, the legacy of fat

«A good way to lose weight is to strip naked and eat in front of a mirror. It always works because almost immediately you are thrown out of the restaurant.»
Boris Makaresko

The first step to hacking habits starts with an act of self-love and begins at the supermarket. Getting your groceries right is good for life and moreover, it makes a difference. Reading a label with the QR Code Reader of your smartphone can help you achieve the best shape.

Cardiovascular problems, hypertension, diabetes, respiratory insufficiency, calculosis, some types of cancer, and atherosclerosis are direct consequences of an inattentive diet that deregulates, through direct inhibition, the tumor suppressor gene P53, which performs, under optimal metabolic conditions Redox reactions, as well as: the removal of DNA fragments, waste, and oxidized neoplastic cells. Notably, is this process is termed «autophagy» and induced after at least 16 hours of fasting. The worrying fact emerging from recent findings is that among the victims of atherosclerosis are increasing numbers of children, in whom the first symptoms of the disease begin to appear between the ages of 6 and 14.

Parents are often misled by poor and incomplete claims, being content to find the calorie or fat content for a given weight listed on the bag of popcorn, not realizing instead that the weight of the package contents is significantly higher and therefore so is the final calorie intake.

From a neuroendocrine perspective, the hypothalamus, pituitary, thyroid, pancreas, and other endocrine glands have for many years been considered a window to be able to analyze proper brain functioning. Some endocrine abnormalities, such as low levels of certain hormones such as estradiol, reduced secretion of luteinizing and follicle-stimulating hormone, and high levels of growth hormone, have been considered as potential causes of eating disorders, but it has also been clarified that for the most part these are consequences of malnutrition rather than pre-existing indicative markers.

Abnormal levels of some neurotransmitters and their respective metabolites, such as norepinephrine and serotonin, which regulate appetite, satiety, and mood, have been shown in the central nervous system and peripheral circulation in patients with eating disorders and in some recovered patients. The serotonergic and noradrenergic systems in patients with bulimia and with anorexia appear to be hypoactive. These levels can be controlled by carrying out a balanced nutritional and physical activity program supported by the intake of suitable amounts of amino acids, vitamins and minerals.

Further investigation is needed into the ways that lead certain genetically predisposed individuals to the onset of eating disorders. The genes incline but do not decide, they say, wanting to imply that a genetic predisposition does not equate to an unbreakable verdict, but only to a tendency that, if properly interpreted will allow one to live a qualitatively perfect existence simply by adapting one's choices to the genetically set path.

BEWARE OF PILLS ON THE WEB!

Consumers, although bombarded by misleading and sometimes fraudulent advertisements, are also to blame. In fact, the number of those who manage to lose weight and retain the result achieved is terribly low, and this simple fact should prompt them to be less «gullible.»

Most of those who, having failed the «diet» road, stubbornly decide not to give up, begin to experiment with alternative therapies. Here then, enter on the scene the «magic» slimming pills, anti-hunger products custom-prepared in pharmacies, or clandestinely imported from countries where they can circulate with the complicity of the Web, which, like a stinging mosquito, targets network users both at home and at work. Among the tons of spam (junk) messages, a good 70 percent involve miraculous tablets for losing weight, while a remaining 30 percent promise incredible potions for experiencing extraordinary sexual performance. A network that makes more money than the drug network.

In the pharmacy things are better, at least you are confronted with a professional. But there were 192,000 deaths in China from counterfeit drugs in 2001 alone, and that is a «government» figure, sure to grow. These fig-

ures should give pause for thought when one considers that about 7 million containers a year arrive in Europe from this country. A small consolation is the fact that our British cousins are not unscathed by this scam epidemic, who have seized 120,000 packages of inauthentic anti-cholesterol tablets in their pharmacies.
Pharmacists are a serious and respected profession, and it is difficult to speculate that one of them might behave dishonestly by buying at lower and advantageous prices, however anything is possible. Sometimes the weak link in the commercial chain are the wholesalers, who by putting thousands of mocked-up boxes into circulation can trigger the release of fake drugs into the circuit, as evidenced by the as many as 93 seizures made in Russia, the 42 in the U.S., the 39 in the U.K., and the 25 in Germany and Israel, just to cite the 2005 Pharmaceutical Security Institute (PSI) top ten. This is an emergency of uncertain but imposing dimensions, ranging in turnover from $3.5 billion, according to FDA (Food and Drug Administration) sources, to an estimated $35 billion from WHO (World Health Organization), which basically means a worldwide average of one in 10 fake pills. These are guideline estimates since, afterall, these are illegal activities, and are clearly difficult to monitor, but nonetheless are extremely profitable.

To form an opinion on the matter, one need only consider that out of every $1,000 invested by criminal organizations, heroin yields nearly $20,000, while on "cheerful" drugs for erectile dysfunction the profit is as high as $500,000, as Mike Chan of the Eli Lilly multinational corporation states: a convenient and profitable business, no doubt, and devoid of significant criminal risks. Thirty years for a kilo of drugs on the one hand, while on the other at most a lecture and a fine...

As far as slimming supplements are concerned, the war is without quarter, and those who enter this jungle of the Web do so at their own peril; although they promise important results for weight reduction, their real efficacy is extremely poor and in any case questionable, when not dangerous and contraindicated. Those who need to lose weight agree to eat a little less, change their lifestyle, and exercise. The achievement of mental and physical well-being is achieved through regular physical activity and proper nutrition-a winning combination.
Find an honest product in a supermarket that proposes a balanced synergy

between physical-imitative activity and a suitable nutritional program, based on balanced meals, supplemented by the proper supply of amino acids, vitamins, and minerals, represents a positive mental approach that finds its proper place in the doctrine of Orthomolecular Biohacking.

GLOBESITY: THE SILENT EPIDEMIC. DEFEAT IT WITH OB

There is a link between chronic diseases and obesity. Obesity is responsible for nearly 60 percent of the 56.5 million deaths per year (45.9 percent of the total global burden of disease). It is safe to say, given the prevalence of obesity in many parts of the world, that we are facing a veritable global epidemic of overweight and obesity, a globesity, as WHO calls it, that is spreading in many countries and may cause, in the absence of immediate action, very serious health problems for millions of people in the coming years.

This is why the WHO has decided to adopt a "Global Strategy on Diet, Physical Activity and Health." Obesity is a chronic disease determined by excess fat mass distributed differently in different body districts and in different individuals.

Obesity "can be treated" but not "cured." With the tools available today, one can easily lose 10 percent of body weight, and it is possible to achieve and maintain this result over time by achieving a substantial lifestyle change.

Chapter 38

Cancer Driver Interception: Ob of Mitochondrial Health

Sweat, O fires to prepare metals, and you, vital irons, be ready, go from Paro to disembowel the mountains to raise kolossal monuments to the king of the Gauls.

(To Louis XIII, 1629, Claudio Achillini)

The new challenge of Orthomomecular Biohacking is to intercept cancer in the bud before it causes irreparable damage. As is known, cancer is one of the main causes of death. In 2020, it was responsible for nearly 10 million deaths worldwide. Lung, colorectal, liver, stomach, and breast cancer accounted for half of these losses, and unfortunately, new diagnoses were common. The new cases were 2.26 million breast cancer, 2.21 million lung cancer, 1.93 million colorectal cancer, 1.41 million prostate cancer, 1.20 million breast cancer skin (non-melanoma) and 1.09 million stomach cancer.

According to Dr Giuseppe Mucci (Founder of the Bioscience Institute, the company with various structures around the world has been a leader in the field of biomolecular tools to evaluate the real state of health of asymptomatic individuals) for the last 40 years, while preventive risk reduction was contributing to the steady decline in death rates from heart disease, cancer has become the leading cause of death in many US states. In 1999, age-standardized heart disease mortality was still higher than cancer mortality in all states, but in 2016 the situation was actually the opposite in 19 states.
Age is among the most important cancer risk factors and the world population is ageing, reaching ages at risk of cancer due to progressive deple-

tion of the pool of available stem cells (see chapter on stem cells).
As is known, stem cells are capable of performing anti-inflammatory, regenerative, revascularizing and paracrine (endocrine modulating) functions.
Imagine them as a precious treasure that has ben given to us at the moment of birth and that we will have to manage with parsimony and foresight throughout our existence by investing it in a correct lifestyle.
Not following the instructions for the use of correct lifestyle habits would be like unexpectedly investing this "bonus vitae" of ours, wasting precious resources of these structural cells (regenerative, revascularizing, hormonal modulating, do you remember?)...
A clear example is that of the physiopathology of the most widespread disease of the dawn of humanity: the "inflammatory intestinal pathology" which involves a large dispersion of stem cells to buffer the rampant inflammation of the digestive mucosa.

THE SHORT BLANKET

If the blanket is short... Learn to curl up!
(ancient Filipino quote)

Like a short blanket, if we squander the few stem cells we have to compensate for bad lifestyles, such as harmful foods intake will lead to digestive inflammation, You bet you'll pay the price like high -interest bank loan
It is not such a good deal to waste our GOLDEN CELLS (our stem cells, author 's note) in the strenuous attempt to neutralize incoming inflammation instead of investing them in solid life-saving actions.
Better save and invest them in regenerative and revascularizing actions credits for our immune capital.
The apparently banal metaphor of the short blanket will help for a better understanding how it is absolutely much more convenient to keep our stem cells without running the risk of remaining metaphorically without them: with our feet uncovered, precisely, exposing us to serious discomfort in the most essential and strategies of our immune defenses, unexpectedly increasing the degenerative and neoplastic risk.
In fact, the improvement in treatment has enormously increased cancer patients lifespan but the cancer risk of survivors is higher which means

that we need to find better targeted therapeutic methods that do not empty these reserves.
In order to make the story short, cancer drugs must not cause a depletion of one's individual "Redox Potential", otherwise the short blanket becomes even shorter.

The endocellular guardians of these precious stem gold reserves are indeed the mitochondria. It is therefore important to keep them dear and if necessary, to curl up so as not to expose our feet.

DISEASES THAT DAMAGE THE MITOCHONDRIA
* Early aging
* Amyotrophic lateral sclerosis (ALS)
* Alzheimer's disease
* Autism
* Cardiovascular disease
* Chronic fatigue syndrome
* Dementia
* Diabetes
* Huntington's disease
* Migraine headache
* Parkinson's disease

ASSOCIATED FACTORS
WITH INCREASE IN MITOCHONDRIAL DAMAGE
* Oxidants leaked while ATP is produced
* Aging (accumulated oxidative damage to mtDNA)
* Genomic susceptibility (especially ApoE4)
* Toxic metals
* Persistent organic pollutants (POPs)
* Many prescription drugs
* Alcohol

NUTRIENTS FOR OB MITOCHONDRIAL:
* β-Oxidation of fats
* FD (riboflavin), NADH (niacin), CoQ10
* Carnitine to transport fatty acids
* Citric acid cycle
* Fe (Iron), magnesium, manganese

  * B1, B2, B3
  * Cysteine (glutathione), lipoid acid)
* ETC
  * CoQ10 (transports high-energy electrons)
  * Riboflavin (complex II)
  * NADH (niacin)
  * Magnesium (final ATP production)

This worsening cancer burden can only be mitigated by an approach in which efforts to treat the disease are accompanied by an increase in its interception. This second route is more cost-effective, has fewer human costs, and will further reduce the burden of cancer on public health and well-being. Today it is possible to shift the focus from early cancer diagnosis and generic reduction of external risk factors to actionable interception of cancer drivers.

Just as we can monitor hypertension, hypertriglyceridemia, obesity and other risk factors that drive the development of cardiovascular diseases, today we finally know that the factors that determine cancer are also measurable.

Everyone can reduce tumor risk by intercepting the "cancer driver", inter-rupting carcinogenesis at any stage prior to the development of an invasive disease, acting on its determining factors.

This is why the assessment of "neoplastic risk" cannot be based exclusively on the clinical history (medical history) and the patient's familiarity. Today the oncogenic risk can be calculated on the basis of objective para-meters, which can be analyzed thanks to modern DNA sequencing techni-ques and identification of the patient's individual biological terrain such as BEV or BTA (BIOELETTRONICA VINCENT, Biological Terrain Asse-sment Vefi Dieta pH - Adolfo Panfili - Ed New Techniques)

We are definitely only looking at the tip of the iceberg of the role of mitochondrial redox dysfunction in human diseases. As the environment becomes more polluted and the prescription of drugs increases, this problem tends to spread, but the good news is that a lot can be done by raising and sharing awareness by spreading this OB manual.

Integr Med (Encinitas). 2014 Apr; 13(2): 8–15. Mitochondria—Fundamen-tal to Life and Health. MD Joseph Pizzorno ND, Editor in Chief)

Early diagnosis can prevent death caused by cancer, but not its onset at the redox (reductive oxide) level.

The primary source of oxidative stress in cells is the loss of oxygen and

high-energy electrons from the mitochondria. This loss increases when key nutrients/protective molecules are missing, such as dose-dependent depletion of CoQ 10 in patients taking statins, a long-known problem, where high-energy electrons are transported between various mitochondrial complexes by CoQ 10. Many factors are associated with increased damage to mitochondria.
(Langsjoen PH, Langsjoen AM. The clinical use of HMG CoA-reductase inhibitors and the associated depletion of coenzyme Q10. A review of animal and human publications. Biofactors. 2003; 18(1–4): 101–111)
Furthermore, primary prevention (i.e. interventions aimed at reducing generic external risk factors such as alcohol, poor nutrition, radiation, smog, metallic excipients of certain drugs, some dental materials, etc.) is often perceived as a passive method that requires deprivation (of smoking, alcohol, some potentially pathogenic foods or substances, etc)
Preventing mortality from cancer means intervening before the biological mechanism is triggered and progressive, essentially to use a rural metaphor: "closing the gates before the oxen have escaped from the fence"...
What would it be like to be able to have a path that even provides for even more timely than early diagnosis of neoplasms, allowing the neoplastic degenerative intention to be intercepted at a cellular biochemical level before it has overflowed the banks of endocellular redox protection. So here is the concept of:

MITOCHONDRIAL HEALTH

A healthy individual at rest produces his body weight in adenosine triphosphate every day!
During maximal effort, this figure can increase by 0.5 to 1.0 kg per minute, which expresses the value of intense metabolic activity.
A large amount of adenosine triphosphate (ATP) must be produced by the mitochondria every second of every day because ATP cannot be accumulated or stored. However, to carry out this intense function, mitochondria hypertrophy their activity, occupying up to 25% of the cellular volume. Cells contain 1000 to 2500 mitochondria.

1 The average cell uses 10 billion ATP per day, which means that a typical adult needs 3.0 × 10 25 ATP (however, the literature on the exact actual ATP requirement for each cell is variable).

2 To maintain this prodigious synthesis the cell's furnace works at very high intensity, so sweat or fires working metals... accomplishing this prodigious feat.
Each mole of ATP must be recycled from ADP 1000 times per day. Since the organism cannot store ATP, the mitochondria must constantly function consistently.
Consider that around 250 g of ATP circulate in cells at any time. That represents about 4.25 watts, the equivalent of the energy of one AA battery.
Every day a healthy person produces 1200 watts!

3 Since the brain uses 70% of ATP, this helps explain the strong correlation between mitochondrial dysfunction and neurodegeneration.

Table 1

Partial list of diseases caused or aggravated by mitochondrial dysfunction

* Premature aging
    • Amyotrophic lateral sclerosis
* Alzheimer's disease
* Autism
    • Cardiovascular disease
* Chronic fatigue syndrome
* Dementia
    • Diabetes
* Huntington's disease
    • Migraine
    • Parkinson's disease

Tapping oncogenic drivers represents an emerging approach to cancer prevention and treatment that aims to identify and target key redox factors of oncogenesis before the development of an invasive, full-blown disease

Here are some key aspects of intercepting cancer drivers:
1. Identification of genetic, epigenetic and environmental factors that drive cancer development.
2. Target precancerous lesions: rather than waiting for the development

of an invasive cancer, cancer driver interception seeks to intercept the carcinogenesis process at the stage of precancerous lesions or tumors at the initial redox (oxidation reductive) stage.

3. Personalized prevention: Intercepting the drivers of cancer involves tailoring prevention strategies to the individual patient, based on their unique genetic and environmental risk factors.

4. Early detection: Interception of cancer drivers highlights the importance of early diagnosis and screening, as detecting and intercepting cancer drivers at an early stage can improve outcomes.

5. Multidisciplinary approach: Intercepting the drivers of cancer requires a multidisciplinary approach that brings together experts in genetics, epidemiology, molecular biology and other fields to develop effective prevention strategies.

Overall, tapping cancer drivers represents a promising new frontier in cancer prevention and treatment, with the potential to reduce cancer incidence and mortality by targeting the root causes of the disease.

In both diagnostics and therapy, medicine has relied less on physical processes and increasingly on chemical processes. Examples in this sense are represented by the clinical chemistry of the medical laboratory and the science of synthetic substances in the chemical and pharmaceutical industry.

With electrochemistry and a more in-depth look at the importance of protons and electrons in vital processes, first the pH value and later also - although initially not considered, the Redox potential were taken to the rank of important diagnostic criteria with the discovery that life is possible only in a delimited pH field, with a precise Redox potential and that even small excursions above or below the normal parameters represent a pathological phenomenon leading to impregnation, degenerative diseases and cancer.
Under the influence of a growing chemical concept, the effects of medicines were considered safe only in the allopathic field and this was until recently.
Successes acquired through the administration of homeopathic remedies were explained nebulously with the concomitant effect of psychic influences induced by the well-known placebo effect. Dilutions beyond the Avo-

gadro or Loschmidt constants were considered as picaresque ironies since the molecules in such preparations could not be measured without even hypothesizing reading scales with excursion ranges different from those in force until then. Today we know about the emission of ultra-weak biophotons also ensured from an experimental point of view, in which the deoxyribonucleic acid DNA or DNS serves at the same time as an accumulator and source of photons. Ultra-weak emission can be physically measured. Photons are the quanta of the electromagnetic field. As biophotons, they are physically effective and biologically active as they are irradiated by organic substances, including foods and medicines. With dissipative structures in the sense of Prigogines and Popp's pharmaceutical effects of a physical nature are created which are maintained in the carrier substance even beyond the Avogadro - Loschmidt constants in the diluent substance, making the aforementioned substances irrelevant.

Already in 1946, the French hydrologist Louis-Claude Vincent supplemented the chemical analyzes of water with physical measurement values. The pH value was already part of the use of water analyses. Vincent completed the chemical analyzes and the pH value with the electrical potential rH2 and the specific resistance r. It was found that the triad pH - rH2 - ro is representative for the quality of drinking water. In the years 1952-53, Vincent managed to find in Lebanon on a large number of patients that the physical or bioelectronic values pH - rH2 - ro are sufficiently representative as a diagnostic tool also for men since the values, depending on how they present, allow recognize a sick organism from a healthy one.

Chapter 39

Health triangle: cancer and degenerative diseases

«When Nero and Agrippina came into conflict,
Seneca approved the execution of the latter as a lesser evil.»

Seneca

The P53 protein, also known as tumor protein 53, is a valuable transcription factor that regulates the cell cycle and serves the function of tumor suppressor. Its activity is critical for ensuring the survival of human beings, and we can evoke its perfect function by following the right lifestyles and activate a strong acid-reduction of the individual biochemical terrain, with particular reference to the function of mitochondria. Mitochondria function by producing energy necessary for the performance of basic endocellular functions. Its function is particularly important in multicellular organisms to suppress nascent tumors; dosing this oncogene is equivalent to dosing the ability to remove tumor waste and toxins from the body.

Comparing the cell to an automobile, it could be said that proto- oncogenes represent the accelerator that, in case of failure, by becoming oncogenic, can careen off the road.

Proto-oncogenes are in fact generally involved in processes controlling cell growth, and in the case of genetic lesions to them, they can become oncogenes, changing their original function and initiating the processes of cancer development.

In some cases, the tumor is caused by an inherited mutation in the proto-oncogene, but much more often mutations are acquired over a lifetime through various cellular processes.

These include what is known as chromosomal rearrangement, which are changes in the structure of chromosomes that lead to changes in the position of parts of DNA. In some cases this rearrangement creates novel combinations, causing the transformation of a proto-oncogene into an oncogene.

In other cases, mutations or gene duplications may arise, leading to continuous activation of certain genes or to the presence in a cell of multiple copies of the same gene.

THE MOST FAMOUS ONCOGENES

The list of known oncogenes is very long and is likely to grow even longer as research progresses. Suffice it to say that in 1989, the year of Bishop and Varmus' Nobel Prize, there were already more than 40 known oncogenes.

To simplify, proto-oncogenes can be divided into categories according to the role they play within the cell and their biochemical properties.

Growth factors (e.g., platelet-derived growth factor; PDGF): stimulate proliferation of target cells.

Growth factor receptors (ERB B, ERB B-2, KIT, MET, RET, ROS, TRK): transmit information across the cell membrane.

Signal transducers (H-RAS, K-RAS, N-RAS, ABL, etc.): help transfer information, for example, from receptors located on cell membranes to the nucleus.

Transcription factors (JUN, FOS, C-MYC, etc.): regulate the expression of target genes or gene families.

Apoptosis regulators (BCL-2): involved in the processes of programmed cell death.

THE ONCO SUPPRESSORS

If oncogenes are the accelerator of the cell, onco suppressors can be compared to brakes.

Onco suppressors or tumor suppressors are genes generally involved in cell division, repair of errors that can be generated in DNA, and the processes of apoptosis (programmed cell death, which is essential to allow the body to stay healthy).

As is the case with oncogenes, onco suppressors can also mutate at some point and lose their braking function, initiating the process of tumor formation.

There is, however, a fundamental difference between oncogenes and onco suppressors: the former become dangerous to the cell when they mutate or by overstimulation are constantly activated, while the latter can give rise to tumors when they are eliminated or inactivated. **The best-known oncosuppressor is p53, which is present in altered form in the largest number of human and other cancers.** The protein produced by this gene was identified in 1979, and for a decade p53 was thought to be an oncogene. It was not until 1989 that researchers reached a breakthrough by coming to the realization that it was actually an oncosuppressor, capable, when unaltered, of defending DNA. Not for nothing can you still read in some textbooks today that p53 is «the guardian of the genome.»

Chapter 40

The analysis of body composition

«Life is measured by deeds and not by days.» Metastasio [Peter Trapassi].

The disposition of fat can be assessed instrumentally, resorting to more or less sophisticated methods to estimate its excess and distribution. These include:

- bioimpedance
- computed tomography
- MRI
- ultrasonography
- plethysmography
- plicometry.

The simplest and therefore most widely used parameter for defining the degree of obesity is the Body Mass Index (BMI or BMI: Body Mass Index), which is derived from the ratio of weight expressed in kilograms to height (in meters)
squared. BMI is a good starting point for beginning to take care of one's health as it represents a trustworthy index for predicting excess fat in the population; however, it should be kept in mind that in the individual and in borderline cases it may underestimate or overestimate body weight. **Weight alone, however, is an incomplete parameter for assessing true body composition because it expresses body mass and not its district composition (ratio of bone, fat, and muscle).** To fine tune this index, one can combine **the measurement of abdominal circumference**, which is a predictive index of abdominal fat, or bioimpedance, which among the

methods is the simplest and most straightforward. Obesity is a complex syndrome that is difficult to classify unambiguously.

For some it is a condition that is associated with metabolic, vascular, and oncological diseases, for others it is a cause of the same. The common orientation is that above a certain body weight it should be considered a chronic condition on par with diabetes and hypertension. It has been demonstrated for years that obese individuals have a qualitatively and quantitatively reduced life expectancy, and therefore the efforts of health professionals must be directed toward finding increasingly efficacious and stable responses.
The prevalence of obesity is increasing in all Western countries, to the point of being defined as an epidemic. In the U.S. it results in 300,000 deaths a year, making it the second leading cause of death after smoking.

Based on the distribution of adipose mass, obesity can be distinguished into:
- android (abdominal)
- gynoid (gluteofemoral)
distinguishable by Waist/Hip ratio (ratio of waist to hip circumference). For the assessment of total body fat on its distribution, plicometry can be used, but it has a high variability depending on the operators.

Skin folds are measured in various anatomic regions, at points where the panniculus adiposus (fat layer) is best represented for that area. Typically, the following are assessed: tricipital plica, bicipital plica, suprailiac plica, subscapular plica.
One of the most widely used methods in recent years for the determination of lipid mass (Fat), lipid mass FFM (Fat Free Mass) and total body water TBW (Total Body Water) is skin bioimpedance analysis (BIA), which uses the bioelectrical impedance provided by the body as an electric current passes through it. Electrical conduction occurs in the presence of water and electrolytes: since almost all of these are contained in the lean mass, BIA can provide an estimate of lean mass, total body water and, by difference, fat mass as well.

OBESITY AND DIABETES

Obesity and Diabetes are two dangerous associated conditions that are unfortunately more common than you might assume; therefore, if you are suffering from one or both of these conditions, this OB manual is definitely for you, working hard to combat these two situations and Getting healthy again. Obesity is less lethal than being underweight, and this, it must be kept under control. After clarifying the causes, you try to change psychosocial conditions and maintain the correct weight, which lowers your cardiovascular risk as you age. There is an insurmountable limit that you will have to respect to enable you to live as healthy and long-lived as possible: let's explore it together.

Obesity (BMI>30 kg/m2) is associated with an increased risk of mortality, this has been known for some time. However, the impact on life expectancy of being overweight (BMI between 25 and 30 kg/m2) was not yet clear. The answer to this question came from the study published by Kenneth Adams et al. of the National Cancer Institute (U.S.) in the New England Journal of Medicine. The prospective study was conducted for 10 years on a sample of more than 500,000 people aged 50 to 70 years and showed a 20 to 40 percent increase in mortality for overweight people. It also confirmed the marked increase in mortality (200-300%) in people with a BMI>30 kg/m2. Another research by a Korean group, published in the same issue of the journal, reached results in line with those in the United States (A. Romero-Corral et al., «Association of bodyweight with total mortality...,» Lancet, 2006; 368: 666-
78). Obesity is generally considered a factor favoring the development of diabetes. U.S. statistical data reveal that 34,413 of the 55,110 deaths that occurred due to diabetes were caused by obesity; epidemiological studies have given a positive answer on the existence of a correlation between the two factors. Genetic studies have pointed out that metabolic alterations present in these individuals have insulin resistance as their first manifestation, even before altered glucose metabolism and weight.

Modern epidemiology has provided a solid answer to this belief: in individuals with a family history of diabetes, BMI is significantly higher than in individuals without a family history. In the Pima Indians, a tribe with a high prevalence of diabetes, a close correlation between familiarity for diabetes and obesity has been demonstrated. In the relationship between diabetes and obesity, it has been observed that the prevalence of diabetes increases consistently with increasing weight and degree of familiarity for diabetes: in E.M. Allen's study, it was seen that, in the partially pancreasectomized dog, concomitantly with the increase in weight diabetes appeared; when the weight was restored to normal, the diabetes disappeared completely.

Chapter 41
Obesity and Biohacking: a practical program

«The sword is more deadly.»
A.P.

The main causes of obesity can be traced back to the following main categories:

- Gender factors (sexuality, etc.);
- Genetic factors (e.g., weight of parents);
- factors that predetermine the ease of fat accumulation and induce alterations in eating behavior and energy expenditure;
- individual anatomy and physiology;
- individual metabolism;
- gestation, birth weight;
- environmental factors;
- Dietary factors: with civilization and the free market there has been a profound qualitative shift in living habits. At the nutritional level, the diet from high carbohydrate-fiber content has shifted toward the excessive introduction of fat. The dietary balance appears dangerously unbalanced. Excess fat certainly makes foods more palatable, but unfortunately for gluttons it results in a clear inhibition of the sense of satiety induced instead by carbohydrate and protein intake;
- Medications that can cause obesity (antipsychotics, antidepressants, antiepileptics, glucocorticoids, insulin, sulfonylureas);
- infections (e.g., adenovirus 36 and six other microorganisms are known to create adiposity);
- Ethno-anthropological and socio-cultural factors;
- Sedentary factor: in Italy, on average, 34% of men and 46% of women

do not engage in any physical activity during leisure time; exercise should be related to the individual's age, but still cannot be excluded from a wellness program. Make a daily appointment with your body;
- Psychological and emotional factors.

There are interactions between factors that further complicate pathogenesis. There are also genetic influences: the probability of becoming obese is five times greater in children whose parents are both obese. Finally, recall selected populations such as the Pima Indians, a tribe with 90% presence of obesity in both sexes. An increase in lipoprotein lipase is found in the obese patient even after slimming, which could be an expression of a primary alteration in adipose tissue.
In nutrition, for the same number of calories, lipids induce greater weight gain than carbohydrates through lower thermo energetic expenditure. Nutrition, through diet quality, can influence the neuroendocrine system with release of neuro-transmitters that act on food intake and appetite: carbohydrates increase brain levels of tryptophan and serotonin; a high-protein meal lowers these levels. Among the peripheral signals that regulate food intake by stimulating the satiety center, the most important are gastric distension, the vagal system, and a number of peptides (glucagon and somatostatin) that can also act via vagal mediation.

The most important hormone recently studied, with regard to satiety, is leptin, a 167-amino acid protein. It is secreted exclusively by adipocytes in response to increased fat mass and is inhibited by insulin and glycocorticoids. This hormone acts at the hypothalamic level where it results in the inhibition of a potent appetite stimulator, neuropeptide Y, and increases the secretion of GLP-1, which is a potent anorectic.

Obesity can be both cause and effect of altered thyroid function. T3-T4-TSH levels are normal under basal conditions and after stimulation with TRH GH levels are reduced both under basal conditions and after provocative stimuli.

AROMATASE, OBESITY, AND MENSTRUAL FLOW

While there may be alterations in the neuroendocrine regulation of gonadal function in both men and women, obese men not infrequently present with sexual dysfunction that can range from mild erectile deficits to more manifest pictures of hypogonadism, with marked reduction in male hormones and the functions they govern.

In obese women, there is a tendency for both hyperestrogenism and hyperandrogenism.

In obese people, basal insulin is elevated and correlates directly with weight. In the face of hyperinsulinemia, basal insulin values are normal with decreased carbohydrate tolerance and thus insulin resistance. In the hyperinsulinemic obese, glucose oxidation and lipogenesis are decreased, while sensitivity to lipolysis inhibition is increased. The latter abnormality may account for reduced hydrolysis of intra-adipocyte triglycerides during fasting.

In fact, in women's adipose tissue, excess estrogens undergo a biochemical transformation (aromatization) with an increase in ovarian estrogens. This results in clinical disorders such as alteration of the menstrual cycle (anorexia, hypooligomenorrhea, functional metrorrhagia) and modest stages of hirsutism, frequently associated with ovarian micropolicystosis, can be found. Obese women are more prone to endometrial carcinoma.

Chapter 42

OB advice to get in shape

«It's not that I'm afraid of dying.
I just wouldn't want to be there when this happens.»

Woody Allen

THE GENES OF OBESITY

A self-respecting biohacker should know about the existence of the obesity gene. For the purposes of weight regulation, the importance of leptin, a hormone that is strategically critical for inducing the sense of satiety and, thus, interrupting food intake, has recently been highlighted. Therefore, one of the most widely accepted hypothesis is that obesity also depends on a deficiency of leptin. Now a study conducted at Beth Israel Deaconess Medical Center in Boston appears to have established a link between lowered leptin levels and a diet low in zinc, a metal found in several foods (lean beef, fish, milk, whole grains). The researchers gave 9 men 30-60 mg of zinc daily for 12 weeks and recorded an increase in hormone levels. On the other hand, switching to a diet low in zinc was noted to reduce leptin levels. As always in these cases, more research and larger samples are needed, but certainly this is consistent with the fact that those on an unbalanced diet are always hungrier than those who eat «properly» (Journal of the American College of Nutrition, 1998; 17: 270-5).
According to research recently published in the journal Annals of Internal Medicine, the tendency to gain weight depends on a gene or, rather, on the DD variant of the Ace (Angiotensin converting enzyme) gene (Strazzullo P. and Siani A., 2005). There would exist genetic factors responsible for overweight and obesity, and this sounds partially consoling for all those who experience guilt and low self-esteem for the failures encountered by trying to follow strict and exaggerated diets, especially in the over-fifties age group.

For more than 20 years, about 1,000 employees of the Olivetti Prospective Heart Study have been kept under observation, and it could be shown that above this age group, subjects with the variant called DD of the ACE genes had a greater tendency to develop overweight with advancing age, due to excess abdominal adiposity and increased «minimum,» or diastolic blood pressure. Singular is the observation that carriers of the DD variant (40 percent of the population) have blood enzyme activity that is about twice that of other individuals; and they are also the ones who gain more weight as they age. Among older patients within the over-53 population, overweight, defined as a body mass index above the conventional limit of 27, was found to be more common in carriers of the DD variant than in the rest of the population: 51 percent versus 36 percent, a statistically highly significant difference. This tendency to be overweight among DD subjects is mainly due to a greater accumulation of fat at the abdominal level. In the group of study participants, it was observed that carriers of the DD variant had over the course of 20 years had 50% more body weight gain than other study participants (on average 4.5 kg versus 3 kg). Furthermore, among those who did not exceed in weight in 1975, the percentage found to be overweight 20 years later was 38 percent in «DD» subjects versus 20 percent in all others. Carriers of the DD variant also showed, over 20 years, a greater increase in diastolic blood pressure, the so-called minimum.
The study is an original contribution to the identification of the genetic factors underlying overweight and obesity, which have also become a serious health threat because they are associated with a very high risk of developing diabetes, hypertension, myocardial infarction, cerebral stroke, osteoarthritis, and some forms of cancer. Based on this phenomenon, an international team of researchers from Imperial College London and colleagues from Hammersmith Hospital in London and the Pasteur Institute in Lille (Public Library of Science Biology, 2003) found that in the complex polygenic association that predisposes to the onset of obesity, another gene in the dock may contribute.

One of these is the GAD2 gene, located on chromosome 10, which appears to contribute to appetite stimulation and more, as a form of it would be prominently associated with obesity by accelerating the production of an amino acid called GABA (gamma-aminobutyric acid). This major brain neurotransmitter exerts inhibitory action on the central nervous system, affecting structures such as the thalamus, amygdala, and putamen nuclei, structural building blocks of the so-called human emotional brain.

→

On their complex correlations and functions depend the emotional, motivational behavior and psychological reinforcement mechanisms (especially those to pleasure and pain) that underlie psychological (especially those to pleasure and pain) that underlie learning processes and the complex mechanism of food gratification.

The cerebral cortex represents the evolutionarily most recent part of the human brain and encompasses the phylogenetically oldest centers of the brain. It integrates and coordinates the functions of all other nerve structures and is the seat of higher psychic functions, such as will, rational intelligence and language. The human brain contains more than 100 billion nerve cells, and each of them connects on average with 50 or 100,000 other neurons. The total number of nerve contacts established in a human brain exceeds that estimated for all the celestial bodies in the universe. This truly astronomical figure can explain the complexity of the functions of this organ in our species, so there is no novelty in noting its involvement with the emotionality of appetite. The moment, in a specific brain area, GABA engages the neuropeptide Y molecule, an appetite stimulus is immediately created in an area called the paraventricular nucleus of the hypothalamus. According to the researchers, this would suggest that all individuals who possess a more active form of the GAD2 gene are likely to accumulate more GABA than normal in the upper hypothalamus brain area. This would explain the triggering of a strong urge to eat with consequent incisive implications in the genesis of obesity. Awareness among physicians and populations in more economically advanced countries has prompted recognition of how necessary it is to prevent obesity; on the other hand, discoveries in molecular biology have increased interest in studying the molecular mechanisms that regulate calorie balance and energy expenditure. Obesity is a genetically «complex» disease in that the genetic factor is not the only one that promotes its development, the environmental component and lifestyle habits are equally important, and it is also «polygenic,» being the result of the activity of dozens, perhaps hundreds, of different genes; therefore, idle no further and as genetics evolves begin to take care of your health.

We are what we eat, and we should carefully select the best foods to consume. This OB manual is designed to increase your health awareness and to make you feel fit, but especially for active prophylaxis of the real tragedy

of this century: cancer. Overexposure to mutagenic agents (primarily smoking and air pollution) but also the abuse of refined and overly high-fat foods has doubled the incidence of cancer in recent decades. It is certain that little can be done against benzene in our cities, much can be done in our own homes for both prophylaxis and treatment of cancers: let us start by following the directions and try not to consume those foods that are responsible for some forms of cancer.
According to the WHO and WFP, it is important to increase the consumption of fruits and vegetables for the prevention of the serious degenerative (noncommunicable) diseases that now afflict the Western world. In this regard, a statement has been drafted that suggests changing dietary habits toward higher intakes of these foods and reducing the consumption of non-organic red meat (Joint WHO/WFP Expert Consultation on Diet, Nutrition and the Prevention of Chronic Diseases, Recommendation 7). WHO and FAO announced the launch of a global initiative to promote fruit and vegetable consumption. Low intakes of fruits and vegetables are a crucial risk factor for diseases such as heart disease, cancer, and obesity, but there is a need to increase the availability of these foods to meet the demands of the world's population. Since the earliest population studies of California Adventists, high consumption of fruits (fresh or dried), tomatoes, and legumes appeared protective against the risk of developing prostate carcinoma (k) (Mills, 1989), and the consumption of animal products and/or obesity were already emerging as risk factors (Snowdon, 1984).

The vegetarian diet, due to its reduced content of fat (however, of plant origin) and calcium and phosphorus, and its intake of substances such as lycopene and phytoestrogens, as well as plant proteins, appears to possess all the requirements for prostate cancer prevention.
The finding has held true over time. In fact, a recent publication (Frazer, 1999) reports that non-vegetarians are more likely to develop prostate cancer.

A diet including adequate fiber intake (with grains, vegetables, legumes and fruits), combined with a reduction in calories and fat, may be one of the possible approaches to the problem of primary and secondary prevention of prostate cancer (Williams, 1999).

In fact, it has been estimated (World Health Report 2002) that low fruit and vegetable consumption is responsible for about 2.7 million deaths a year, placing it among the top 10 risk factors for death. The announcement was made in Rio de Janeiro, Brazil, at the annual meeting of the WHO Global Forum for the Prevention and Control of Noncommunicable Diseases. «There is strong and growing evidence that adequate intakes of fruits and vegetables help prevent many diseases and can promote better health, but most of the world's population consumes too little of them,» Pekka Puska, WHO Director for Noncommunicable Disease Prevention and Health Promotion, said in Rio.

It has recently been discovered in some vegetables (especially tomatoes), the presence of lycopenes, molecules that are capable of blocking the rampant genes capable of triggering carcinogenic mutations. Here is a reflection on how many people, sidetracked by silly fads of false medicine, have eliminated tomatoes from the diet because they are (according to them) allergenic foods. Food allergies in general are very rare and tomatoes are among the foods least responsible for allergies. When a tomato generates allergic reactions, this is probably due to overuse of pesticides with which the plant has been treated. Eat lots of tomatoes, then, but only in season and sun-ripened. Never eat an out-of-season vegetable or fruit.

Non-communicable diseases are responsible for about 60 percent of global deaths and 45 percent of the global disease burden. Unhealthy diets, along with the Sedentary lifestyle and tobacco abuse are among the critical preventable risk factors of noncommunicable diseases. Adequate daily intakes of fruits and vegetables are likely to contribute to the prevention of major noncommunicable diseases such as cardiovascular disease, type 2 diabetes, obesity, and certain cancers such as prostate in men, breast in women, and lung in both sexes, although with greater prevalence in men. **The recently published report of the WFP/WHO Committee of Experts on Diet, Nutrition and Prevention of Infectious Diseases recommends a minimum intake of 400 g of fruits and vegetables per day (excluding starchy tubers such as potatoes) for the prevention of chronic diseases**, including heart disease, cancer, type 2 diabetes and obesity. Intake of a wide variety of fruits and vegetables helps ensure adequate intakes of many micronutrients, dietary fiber and a large amount of beneficial non nutrients, the two international agencies say. Increased intakes of fruits and vegetables also help limit high intakes of foods high in fat, sugar and salt.

The pharmacy of the plant world is a minimally explored treasure chest of health that is increasingly full of surprises. Much hope would be pinned on the use of aloe, which an Israeli doctor has reportedly been using for years as an anti-cancer therapy; we personally cannot ratify this as we have no specific experience in this regard. Striking results, however, we have been able to see on inflammatory skin conditions even in combination with common drugs, in intestinal dysbiosis and in headaches. Also in the field of medicinal plants, the antioxidant power of green tea has been known for centuries and could exert an interesting action against tumors, although further confirmatory studies are needed on catechins (active components of green tea), true life-saving molecules.

Chapter 43
Low cholesterol and black mood

*«Don't let medical and political authorities mislead you.
Inform yourself about the reality of the facts and decide for yourself how to live a happy life and how to take action to improve the world.»*
Linus Pauling

Cholesterol is not a criminal! Sure, it should be kept at «normal» levels and controlled, but without over-restricting, since low blood cholesterol at a certain age can open the door to depression. The warning comes from the Division of Epidemiology at the University of California at San Diego, which (in a sample of more than 1,000 men aged 50 to 89) found that «black humor» is three times more common in people with low circulating cholesterol. Low levels of this parameter in the blood can trigger depression has already been suggested by the increased cases of suicide found among people who have undergone treatment pharmacological and to unbalanced diets.

REJUVENATE ARTERIES AND AVOID BYPASS

Unless one is faced with hereditary or familial disorders of lipid metabolism, drugs termed «cholesterol-lowering» that profoundly alter bile fluid density, predisposing to the occurrence of lithiasis (stones) of the intra and extrahepatic biliary tracts, are definitely contraindicated. Maintaining «safe» cholesterol levels can be pursued and maintained simply by observing an adequately normocaloric diet without excess animal fats (NEFA) in conjunction with the administration of natural L-tocopherol 1200 I.U./day. In addition, many scholars recommend the use of L-carnitine at dosages between 1500-3000 mg/day to improve fatty acid oxidation, especially at the myocardial level, in subjects with angina pectoris and coronary insufficiency. It is useful to supplement with L-taurine intake

in the order of 2 g/day in order to facilitate the flow of potassium and calcium ions into cardiac cells.
Subjects who can be successfully treated with the aid of the orthomolecular approach are adults of both sexes at moderate or high vascular risk, monitored for cholesterolemia at least annually, except for those pre existing diseases (hypothyroidism, nephrotic syndrome, dysproteinemia, diabetes mellitus, obstructive liver disease) that are possible causes of hypercholesterolemia. On the other hand, situations of mild hypercholesterolemia, without familiarity with specific vascular or endocrine diseases, do not require specific treatment other than dietary treatment.
In 1910, Nobel Prize winner Alexis Carrel showed that human beings live just over 50 percent of their actual life potential. «We are genetically programmed for a life span of 120 years», Russian scientists also confirm. The decrease in life expectancy is related to the aging of arteries due to excess calcium accumulating in them. Excess circulating calcium in our blood released to buffer situations of excessive tissue acidification can cause degenerative diseases such as atherosclerosis, heart disease, diabetes, cancer, ischemic attacks, cirrhosis, kidney disease, aging, etc., and diseases resulting from the thickening and hardening of arterial vessels. It is certainly possible to live longer and more actively simply by using vitamin C as a supplement.
When arteries narrow, blood flow to cells, tissues, and organs decreases significantly. **In twenty-four hours, more than 5 trillion cells are completely replaced by blood supply.** The replacement of structural material allows vital tissue activity to be maintained. If blood circulation is compromised, these processes become discontinuous and the compromised area of the body stops functioning. This is the mechanism of the onset of hardening and aging of the arteries.
The administration of inorganic minerals, often administered in megadoses, «administered by profusion,» through self-styled nutritional pseudo-protocols, results in an overload of electrolytes in the blood, which tend to congest renal filtration because, in the long run, they result in substantial limestone deposition, which in turn disturbs the normal secretion of the nephron (filtering unit of the kidney), which loses its normal function by opening access to degenerative and cancer diseases. The only form of calcium that can be administered is organic calcium from the plant world, or in the form of amino chelate, hydroxyapatite, etc.
Be careful, however, because excessive calcium intake may be worse than initial deficiency itself, facilitating the onset or worsening of arterial steno-

sis (coronary, cerebral, etc.), biliary-renal lithiasis, and atherosclerosis. Prominent scientists currently recognize that the main causes of alterations in the circulatory system are precisely spasm or constriction of the arteries and, although the cause has not yet been perfectly identified, a large amount of calcium is deposited with consequent, progressive reduction in the diameter of the vessels causing atherosclerosis affecting the middle tunica of the arterioles, resulting in loss of musculature and inability to contract and dilate. The former mechanism intervenes in 99% of cases, the latter, of course, in 1%. The cell, poorly supplied with blood because of stenosing lesions to the lumen of the arteries, undergoes a series of degenerative phenomena, among which the one currently receiving the most interest concerns the alteration of calcium metabolism.
This is normally an extracellular ion that, under conditions of tissue ischemia, bursts within the cytoplasm, disrupting the limiting membrane and destroying the cytoskeleton, preventing normal exchanges with the surrounding tissue and replacing other cytoplasmic elements. The cell thus affected is left with no choice but to make all remaining energy reserves available in order to remove the abnormal accumulation of calcium created in it. Progressive deterioration ensues, often irreparably damaging the intima of the arteries.

IDEAL WEIGHT AND ABSTRACT WEIGHT

Recently, the WHO has set new criteria for classifying obesity on the basis of BMI, (kg/m2): a value of 24.9 has been set as the upper limit of normality, while grade I, II and III obesity has been defined as those BMI values between 25 and 29.9, between 30 and 39.9 and greater than 40, respectively. That said, it should be emphasized that the message to be conveyed is to aim for a realistically achievable goal: one should aim not to achieve the so-called ideal weight, an abstract number and expression of calculations that have only statistical value, but the so-called reasonable weight, meaning, by that term, the weight maintained effortlessly after the age of 21 and allowed good physical, mental and social health.
It has now been widely demonstrated that a reduction of 10 to 15 percent of initial weight is sufficient to induce significant improvements in hypertension, diabetes, and cardiovascular disease. If you are severely obese and your BMI exceeds the guideline value of 30, before embarking on any physical activity program you would do well to consult your medical professional since the diagnosis of grade II and III obesity is generally clinical, and in addition to performing common routine examinations it would be helpful to assess your BMI with them.

It will be your primary care physician who will confirm the need for laboratory tests (both genetic and endocrinological), which should be prescribed only if clinical symptoms become evident that necessitate the differential diagnosis with genetic and endocrine obesity. In individuals with essential obesity, to determine whether overweight-related complications have already been established, it is recommended to perform:

Lipid screening:

total cholesterol,

HDL cholesterol ("good" cholesterol),

LDL cholesterol;

comprehensive urine examination;

Basal blood glucose and insulinemia or possibly oral glucose loading test with assessment of blood glucose and insulinemia (glucose tolerance test);

liver function;

if hepatomegaly and/or hypertransaminasemia is found, in-depth liver function tests and liver ultrasound;

electrocardiogram;

Any in-depth cardiological investigations;

if high blood pressure values are found, serious blood pressure checks; if blood pressure does not normalize after weight loss, further diagnostic investigation is recommended;

Sleep polygraphic study if history suggestive of sleep apnea.

Obesity, fat mass distribution and genetic make-up

Obesity and adipose mass distribution are controlled by genes that play a decisive role in the mechanisms that modulate their development, according to the journal Proceedings of the National Academy of Sciences, which describes work done by researchers at the Joslin Diabetes Center, who used sophisticated genetic diagnostic techniques for the first time to understand how genes may control the development of fat cells in the abdomen and epidermis, respectively.

By analyzing a person's genetic make-up, it is currently possible to determine whether he or she is obese and how fat will be distributed in his or

her body (C. Ronald Kahn et al. at the Joslin Diabetes Center at Harvard Medical School). It has also long been known that in other animal species genes play an essential role in body development, and it is genes that determine the morphogenesis of organs such as the head, tail, and wings. No surprise then that **humans genes determine the amount of fat cells and their distribution.** As is well known, in obesity the location of body fat can significantly influence the risk of developing chronic diseases.
The team of researchers examined the genetic makeup of fat cell samples taken from the surface of internal organs or the subcutaneous area of laboratory mice and about 200 normal to obese patients (both abdominal and subcutaneous obesity individuals present). Theorizing that fat cell distribution patterns, and perhaps obesity itself, may originate from genes implicated in the control of body development, the researchers found that 12 genes involved in development play an important role in the process of fat deposition, and at least three of these appear to be somehow related to obesity. By comparing the activity of these three genes (Tbx15, Gpc4, HoxA5) in fat samples taken from patients with normal body weight and from overweight or obese patients, the researchers found marked differences. «The expression of the genes tested was so diverse,» explains Stephane Gesta, one of the team's researchers, «that we were able to identify the BMI and waist-to-hip ratio WHR of the overweight population simply by studying the expression level of these genes. This suggests to us that their activity is certainly related to the pathogenesis of obesity. This may be a process that begins at very early stages of life.» (Source: Joslin Diabetes Center press release, 2006).

Chapter 44
OB Tips to be Fit: Stop osteoporosis with diet and physical activity

«How to reach a goal? Unhurriedly but relentlessly.»
Goethe

Osteoporosis is a disease that affects the skeleton, characterized by increased bone fragility caused by loss of bone strength and thickness. It is also called the silent disease, as it is often not diagnosed until one suffers a fracture, usually after a fall. **Osteoporosis affects more than 3 million Italian women, a social disease with a devastating impact, for which necessary medications should be free even for those who have not yet suffered a fracture.** In Italy, osteoporosis afflicts one-third of women between 60 and 70 and two-thirds of those over 80, causing more deaths than some cancers. In the EU alone, about 400.000 women suffer osteoporosis-related hip fractures each year. IOF estimates that it will be one million by 2050. Not only that, 24% of those who have suffered multiple fractures are at risk of death within a year; 10% die immediately and 28% can no longer live independent. In Italy, the NHS spends 619 million euros solely on the treatment of femur fractures, and osteoporosis drugs are reimbursable only for those who have already suffered a fracture. It has been argued that osteoporosis is a disease that generally shows up in old age, but has its roots in the age of development: a lack of «saturation» of bone tissue in the first 20 years of life will condition the development of the disease in the years of old age. Such saturation of mineral salts such as calcium, phosphorus, etc., is clearly influenced by the type of diet followed in the first two decades of life. The osteoporosis problem is of global significance: the significant increase in the average lifespan of the population highlights pathologies that, in a time even recently, did not stand out in all their current drama. Ever since Albright defined «osteoporosis» in 1941 as a condition in which bone mass was deficient, characterized by an increased «radiolucency» of the spine and, from a clinical point of view, an increased number of fractures, there has been a need to quantify this skeletal «weakness,» this lack of mechanical strength. Today it is finally possible. In fact, we have trustworthy machines and the cost of the examination is relatively inexpensive.

The ESOPO study is the first epidemiological survey on the prevalence of osteoporosis in Italy. It collected clinical data from 16,000 subjects through 83 specialist centers distributed throughout the country, highlighting that osteoporosis is an under-diagnosed and under-treated disease. About 23 percent of women after the age of 40 and 14 percent of men over the age of 60 have the disease, while in the same age groups osteopenia affects 42 percent of women and 34 percent of men.

Women, as a result of the drastic drop in estrogen after menopause, are much more vulnerable than men, with an almost four times higher risk of developing this condition. However, osteoporosis remains linked to many factors specific to aging and, given Italy's demographic trends, is likely to become increasingly common.

It is well known that postmenopausal female subjects are affected in most cases. The depletion of bone mass sometimes progresses irreversibly, leading to clinical pictures of severe impairment, necessitating assistance and expensive nursing care for many years.

CONSUME ORGANIC SOY TO SLOW DOWN AGING

The intake of non-genetically modified soy-derived proteins that provide soy isoflavones is provided and recommended in this manual. These substances are valuable for health in general, and particularly for that of menopausal and postmenopausal women, conferring valuable benefits to the osteoarticular and urogenital systems. (Eden J., Knight D., Mackey R., Hormonal effects of isoflavones, Frank Rundle House, Royal Hospital for Women, Paddington, N.S.V. 2021, Australia; M. Ruiz- Larrea et al: Antioxidant activity of phytoestrogenic isoflavones; Free Rad Res., 1997, 26, 63-70; G. Kukreja, Dietary soybean protein prevents bone loss in an ovariectomized rat model of osteoporosis).

Soybean is a legume native to Central Asia, where it has been cultivated for more than five thousand years. It has virtually no issues with cultivation, grows well at different altitudes, and is resistant to frost, drought and disease. The plant produces seeds valuable for their high nutritional value, from which a wide variety of preparations have been obtained, either as foods or as dietary supplements.

Its composition: isoflavones and related glycosides, genistein, daidzein, glycitein, saponins, lecithin.

Its properties: soybeans that contain a particular family of phytoestrogens called «isoflavones.»

In addition to being a protein-rich food, soy is a food through which our health can improve. In fact, it reduces the risk of breast cancer, heart disease, osteoporosis, menopausal symptoms, diabetes, kidney problems, and other chronic diseases. The fact that Japanese women suffer less frequently from some forms of cancer (breast, uterus, ovarian) than Western women, and also have reduced menopausal symptoms, particularly hot flashes, could be attributed to their soy-rich diet (they consume 25 to 45 mg of soy isoflavones daily). Studies in other populations show that 40 percent of women on a diet rich in soy isoflavones have a decreased incidence of skin rashes and hot flashes.

The isoflavones contained in plants have the primary function of antioxidants, in that they protect against ultraviolet radiation and other sources of free radicals. Isoflavones, when taken with soy-rich foods, function as both antioxidants and phytoestrogens, providing tremendous benefits; in fact, female estrogen (the female sex hormone), partially protects against heart disease and osteoporosis. Estrogen circulating in the bloodstream has a certain affinity with certain tissues in certain organs, to which it binds through receptors, somewhat like what happens with the key that enters the keyhole, opening it and allowing it to enter the desired environment.

Tissues that contain receptors for estrogen binding are in the breast, vagina, and uterus; when the receptor binds with estrogen, it sends a message to the tissue and it begins to grow. This is normal during certain times of life (e.g., during pregnancy), but at other times it can increase the risk of cancer, and therefore it is critical to have a balanced amount of estrogen.

In soybeans, the predominant isoflavones are two: **genistein** and **daidzein**, both with antioxidant properties. Genistin is the radical deactivator, and being unbound, is more potent, while daidzein has more modest antioxidant activity. Since it is scientifically known that certain types of cancers are a result of non-genetic factors, such as diet, lifestyle, environmental pollution, etc., following a proper diet low in saturated fat and rich in vitamins (A, C, beta-carotene, E), selenium, fiber, amino acids, minerals and nutrients in the right balance can reduce the predisposing factors for cancer occurrence.

Soy isoflavones, in addition to having phytoestrogenic and antioxidant actions, help prevent angiogenic processes (vessel formation) where the tumor is developing, and also act in an inhibitory sense on enzymes responsible for tumor growth.

ISOFLAVONES AND MENOPAUSE

The first symptoms of menopause occur when the ovaries begin to slow estrogen production. Without estrogen production, which stimulates ovulation, menstrual flow is ceases.
Menopause is a natural process and should not be considered a disease. Like a season, menopause begins with a range of symptoms, many of which can be attributed to hormonal change. Some of these, such as vaginal dryness, are attributable to estrogen deficiency or complete absence; others, such as hot flashes, are caused by changes in multiple hormonal systems.
Generally, a therapy based on combining an estrogen with another hormone called progestin is administered to combat these symptoms. This therapy serves, no doubt, to combat hot flashes, but it can lead to the onset of dangerous side effects among which the possible increased risk of developing forms of breast and uterine cancer should be noted.
A natural alternative to the use of hormonal drugs, which is completely risk-free, is a diet rich in soy isoflavones, which can provide the right amount of phytoestrogens, similar to synthetic estrogen. In post-menopausal women, in addition to low estrogen levels, there is increased bone calcium loss and the development of osteoporosis. Traditional pharmacotherapy in these cases involves calcium administration combined with hormone therapy.

SOY AND THE CARDIOVASCULAR SYSTEM

Generally, it is the male sex that has greater cardiovascular vulnerability, while women are more susceptible to this disease after the menopausal period, when their natural biological estrogen protection drops.
Because estrogens protect against heart attacks, when their circulating blood concentrations decrease there is a decrease in HDL in the blood and a consequent increase in LDL, which tends to promote the onset of heart disease. In addition, amino acids in soy protein, essentially L-glycine and L-arginine, keep insulin levels in the body low, thus decreasing the amount of cholesterol synthesized (A.L. Murkies et al.: «Dietary flour supplementation decreases post-menopausal hot flushes: Effect of soya and wheat»

Maturitas, 21 (1995), 189-195; H.Adlercreutz: «Is genistein the key to soy's success?», Lancet, 1992, 16 (339), 1233).

The antioxidants contained in isoflavones are equally important in the cardiovascular preventive arena with regard to the prevention of coronary heart disease, due to the significant supply of antioxidants that neutralize circulating free radicals. Also important in soy is the intake of folic acid, which, among other things, is found in abundance in certain foods such as green leafy vegetables (spinach, broccoli, asparagus, lettuce), oranges (and orange juice from concentrate), legumes, cereals, and in fruits such as lemons, kiwis, and strawberries. The cooking process, however, destroys much of the folate in foods. Folic acid (folate) is vitamin B9; it is not produced by the body, but must be taken in through food and intestinal bacterial flora; the daily requirement under normal conditions is about 0.2 mg. In recent decades, folic acid has been recognized as essential in the prevention of neonatal malformations, particularly those affecting the neural tube, which originates in the early stages of embryonic development. During pregnancy, therefore, folate requirements double to 0.4 mg because the fetus utilizes maternal reserves.

Although its role is not known in detail, vitamin B9 is essential for DNA and protein synthesis and the formation of hemoglobin, and it is particularly important for tissues undergoing processes of proliferation and differentiation, such as, precisely, embryonic and bone tissues. Its presence lowers levels of the amino acid Homocysteine, which is associated with the risk of cardiovascular disease and myocardial infarction. In the formation of bone texture, the presence of vitamins B6 and B9 is relevant, as these are necessary for the body to convert the amino acid methionine to cysteine. In case of deficiency, there will be an increase in homocysteine, which is known to be implicated in the genesis of osteoporosis through the interference carried out by this compound on the regular lattice arrangement of collagen fibers. Folic acid, in the presence of the vitamins mentioned above, lowers homocysteine levels.

Toxicological studies confirm that soy extracts have no primary or secondary toxicity at recommended doses, neither in the short nor long term, making the use of isoflavones an ideal solution for improving dietary quality. The possible use of soy isoflavones in the prevention of certain cancers (breast, endometrial, prostate, and colon) is currently being investigated; some applications have already been reported at the 2nd International Symposium on the Role of Soy in the Prevention and Treatment of Chronic Diseases.

THE ADVANTAGES OF GOOD HABITS

In conclusion: physical activity, which is physiological in children, should be a part of daily life at any age, of course if there are no current pathologies such as to contraindicate it. It, combined with hygienic rules of life (diet and smoking above all), should not turn everyone into a marathon runner. Low-intensity activity, but with constant commitment, such as a «jog» of no more than an hour, three times a week, is sufficient. In the ideological sphere, as well as in other age groups, countless benefits can be pursued with methodical and efficacious training:

greater strength;

1) Increased resistance to stress;
2) Increased resistance to fatigue;
3) Better tendency for psychic relaxation;
4) Better sleep;
5) Sociality and new friendships;
6) improved muscle tone;
7) help in burning calories, losing weight or keeping fit;
8) Aid in appetite control;
9) Reduction in LDL cholesterol and triglycerides, improved carbohydrate tolerance;
10) increased HDL cholesterol;
11) Reduction in blood pressure values both at rest and under effort;
13) Decreased heart rate both at rest and under stress;
14) According to numerous studies, total mortality and cardiovascular mortality are reduced by 25% in well-trained subjects.

About three-fourths of the calories we take in are used by the body for its basic needs, about one-fourth is used for physical activity; increased exercise promotes extra calorie consumption. Should dynamic walking not be to your liking, keep in mind that it would be beneficial to exercise at least three times a week to improve cardiovascular fitness and vary the duration of exercise from 20 to 40 minutes. Exercise sessions should last no more than an hour, after an initial 10-minute warm-up period, with light exercises to avoid muscle stretching and allow a gradual increase in heart rate. The most common risk in exercise is from muscle or joint injuries. For untrained people and especially for heart patients, it is necessary to refer to specialized rehabilitation centers in order to follow an individualized and well-defined training program, so as to limit as much as possible the risks of poorly adapted training.

Chapter 45
Lamark was right: function develops the organ!

«Function develops the organ, so in order to function you have to move, both intelligently and daily.»
A.P.

Participating in some physical activity on a regular basis serves to instruct the nervous system to cultivate tissues, organs, bones and muscles and keep them efficient and healthy. The concept of «relatively stable» perhaps requires some clarification. Let us compare different bodily functions: for example, learning, which is primarily related to brain function, is relatively very stable function; in fact, what is learned (studied and learned!) remains in the mind for years and years, although obviously something is forgotten; moreover, what is learned at a young age remains well imprinted in the mind. Let us now consider cardiovascular and muscular function: compared to brain function, heart and muscles forget more easily what they have learned. Again, however, if heart and muscles are stressed when young, it is better. It is obvious that all those who do not practice physical activity will feel their hearts in their throats when quickly climbing stairs, but even those who have some familiarity with sports can clearly recognize when they are well or poorly trained in climbing them. In fact, it only takes a few weeks of inactivity to realize this; finally, it is well known to all the staggering training load that Olympic athletes undergo to improve performances and records. What happens to them when they give up competitive activity? It is very simple: they become like others, and this is because, over the years, their muscles and heart slowly forget. Perhaps the brain forgets less because it is practically in use all the time, and if this is a convincing explanation, then it is reasonable to suggest that everyone should practice some physical activity with continuity. In summary, memory, even muscle memory, should always be cultivated. Taking up the comparison with the brain, it can be said: the function of learning is guided by a teacher, a professor, and physical activity may also need the same support, hence the decisive role of the personal trainer (PT). Moreover, medical science agrees on at least one point: «The risks associated with practicing sports are far less than those of not practicing them.»

HORMESIS AND OB: GAMBLING WITH STRESS

Stress expresses the power of life and is synonymous with change. Stress is a typical adaptive reaction of the body to a generic physical or psychic change. Humans follow cycles: relaxation, alarm state, tension and reaction to the alarm situation.

Everyone experiences and somaticizes stress in a personal and unique manner, but the adaptive roots of cellular biochemistry that characterize it are common. What is poison for some may be panacea or elixir of life for others. Only the substrate on which the seed of stress is sown changes. For stress is influenced by the intervention of our thoughts. Everyone, in the presence of a stressful situation, produces disparate thoughts and thus different emotions and behaviors.

Thus stress can also be aggravated by a subjective and highly personal reinterpretation of reality mediated by specific anatomical structures such as the amygdala, rhinencephalon, hippocampus, etc. Such organs of the central nervous system are capable of processing and amplifying meanings and consequences of stressful experience, even aggravating or exacerbat-ing the connotation of each individual's responses.

What causes stress?

The body reacts to stress by increasing the secretion of certain hormones and inhibiting others. Stress causes physical changes in the brain and body. Fatigue, anxiety, depression, and sleep disorders are caused by chemical malfunctions in the brain. Prolonged stress can cause physical damage. It is possible to give an example score to stress, not so much to trivialize its contents to simple numerical entities, but rather to visualize its scale of intensity and consequent impact in daily life (see table). Messenger sub-stances such as serotonin, norepinephrine, and dopamine are among the main chemicals that begin to malfunction. Stress can cause poor produc-tion of these substances. Serotonin is important for sleeping well, for reg-ulating our internal clock, for regulation of body temperature, by the contraction of smooth muscles of the vessels, intestines, bronchi, uterus, and bladder, in the regulation of intestinal automatism, in the modification of blood pressure; intervenes in allergic and inflammatory processes, reduces bleeding time, determines migraine symptomatology, etc. Serotonin is also converted to melatonin and vice versa.

The stress evaluation scale (Holmes and Rahe, 1967)

EVENT	VL	EVENT	VL
Death of spouse	100	Removal from a child's home	29
Divorce	73	Problems with in-laws	29
Separation	65	Outstanding personal achievement	28
Period of imprisonment	63	Wife's commencement or termination of employment	26
Personal injury or illness	53	Start or end of school	26
Wedding	50	Changes in living conditions	25
Dismissal	47	Review of personal habits	24
Reconciliation with spouse	45	Problems with superiors	23
Retirement	45	Change in working hours and conditions	20
Changes in the health of a member of the family	44	Change of residence	20
Pregnancy	40	School change	20
Sexual difficulties	39	Change in sleeping habits	19
Increase in household size	39	Change in religious activities	19
Business restructuring	39	Change in social activities	18
Changes in financial status	38	Small loan or mortgage	17
Death of a close friend	37	Change in sleep habits	16
Transition to another type of work	36	Change in the number of family meetings	15
Change in the frequency of marital quarrels	35	Change in eating habits	15
Mortgage or lease of high magnitude	3	Vacations	1
Inability to take out a loan or mortgage	30	Christmas period	12
Changing professional responsibilities	29	Violations of the law of moderate severity	11

BIORHYTHMS: REGULATING THE STRESS CLOCK

There is a science that studies the intercurrent relationships between atmospheric-meteorological phenomena and human biological phenomena: chronobiology. When is it best to exercise? Granted that the answer is still subjective and therefore variable, one cannot be categorical and inflexible, although it is advisable to do it in the morning if possible. Some individuals «burn» best in the morning as soon as they get up- Blood Group A people. Others in the afternoon-evening: blood group 0 individuals. - When they have filled up with energy and feel charged having the need to also discharge the tensions accumulated during the day (see *The Blood Group Diet*, New Techniques). Working out at the wrong time can aggravate overall fatigue, and you know how important it is not to bingo with stress. Choose the golden moments of your day well to get rid of your burdens because the body reacts differently depending on the times of day at which a given activity is performed.

Chronobiology and rhythms of life

Chronobiology, from the Greek chrónos 'time' and from biology, is a branch of biology that studies periodic phenomena in living organisms and their adaptation to relative solar and lunar rhythms.

Circadian rhythm: this is the periodicity with which the maximum daily resources are available.

Ultradian rhythm: is that less than 20 hours (e.g., the sleep phase).

Circalunar rhythm: this is the one corresponding to the 4-week lunar synodic rhythm. Arrhenius, in 1898, in his paper entitled Cosmic Influences on Physiological Phenomena, claimed the existence of lunar influence on births, deaths, seizures and menstrual flow in women. In Newton's theory, the gravitational interaction between the Moon and the Sun on the water mass of the seas induces a periodic, regular and constant oscillation that involves in the course of the lunar day (duration of 24 hours and 50 minutes) two rises and two falls. It is permissible to consider tides as extended waves with a period of 12 hours and 25 minutes, or 44,676 seconds.

For the thermal convection of huge air masses, the dynamics of the tides involve large variations in atmospheric pressure. The rhythm of the human respiratory rate is the harmonic of the tidal wave, being in clear resonance with it, as can be inferred from the fact that the period of respiratory acts is 13,000 times smaller than that of the tides: 44,676: 13,000 = 3.43 seconds.

→

Similarly, the dynamics of blood fluids in the human body seem to resonate with the syzygial rhythm of the tides. In fact, it turns out that, as a result of the displacement of huge masses and volumes of water, tidal currents develop in the seas, the forward speed of which would be about 0.5 m/s, corresponding to the speed of blood flow within arterial and venous vessels (10 cm/s in veins and 20-40 cm/s in arteries).

Since women's bodies are richer in water than men's, they will respond like the oceans more sensitively to the changes in gravitational attraction found during the lunar synodic month, creating the cyclical pattern of menstrual flow. It is not coincidental, therefore, that a woman's menstrual cycle has the same duration as the lunar cycle, or about 29 1/2 days. The duration of gestation corresponds to 9 lunar months (the nine morphologically closely resembles the figure of a fetus in the womb), or 265.8 days, according to a study performed in 1959 by Menaker on a sample of 250,000 births. The process of reproduction would also be marked by astronomical rhythms external to the intrinsic biology of the human cell. The changing position of the Moon relative to the Sun is also responsible for changes in the environment and behavior that have been known for centuries. The irregularity of cycles in many cases may be correlated with exposure to light during the night, that is, with an incorrect synchronization of the circadian secretory rhythm of melatonin with the full moon phase. Women suffering from dysmenorrhea, simply by turning on low lux lights during the night of the 14th-15th-16th day can regularize their flow without resorting to medication. Simple coincidence or obvious observation that the physiological functions of the human organism resonate with the vital, pulsating activity of the Earth understood as a living organism. Each organ or apparatus, each innermost cell has a very precise and physiological «calibration» that is approximately almost monthly.

Monthly biorhythms

The main monthly biorhythms are different in nature:
physics (23 days)
emotional (28 days)
intellectual (33 days).
The craftsman who meticulously tares the human biological clock is the hypothalamus, located at the base of the skull in the button room, which it shares with its superior in rank, the pituitary gland.

The circadian rhythm

This rhythm is the one that most concerns this program. The functions that interact with the daily (circadian) rhythm are diverse and affect all the natural and physiological processes of our body, where we reach a greater peak with regard to the level of attention, dexterity and motor co-ordination, body temperature (e.g., the minimum seems to be around 6 a.m. and the maximum around 4 p.m.). **During the day there is also a variation in hormone production and thus strength, glycogen stores, respiratory stages, blood fluids, and of course also at the level of the central nervous system.**

Think of a workout performed after one or more sleepless nights: I challenge anyone to give their best and feel good! In addition to the disruption of physiological processes, a stressful situation would occur that would make training not only more strenuous, but fundamentally fruitless. Lack of rest at night interferes with the nervous and musculoskeletal system's ability to respond and recover, with accumulation of toxic waste (ammonium, see *Orthomolecular Medicine: a human-friendly therapy*, New Techniques) and loss of fine motor coordination resulting in loss of precision in movements, slowing down and greater energy expenditure.

Overdoing it makes training counterproductive. Keep in mind, however, that according to recent studies:

- reaction time to visual or auditory stimuli has a peak between 4 and 6 p.m. at maximum body temperature values. It is said that for every degree centigrade increase in temperature, nerve conduction velocity increases by 2.4 m/s;
- a highest level of cognitive ability and intellectual work, as well as the precision of gesture, is recorded in the morning;
- explosive strength and maximal strength present the highest level in the period between 4pm and 6pm;
- Metabolic capacities, both aerobic and anaerobic, are highest in the late afternoon when maximum values of oxygen consumption (VO2max), lung ventilation, systolic output, and cardiac output are noted. In this phase of the day, it would result;
- higher athletic endurance by performing constant work at high intensity, as well as the ability to produce lactic acid.

The factors that influence circadian rhythms are mainly external, the most important being the alternation of day and night. Not surprisingly, most human activities take place as long as there is light and stop when the sun goes down. We have evidence of this biological clock when we have to

move to a place where there is a different time zone, especially if it is 10-12 hours.
Automatically, and quite naturally, this particular clock will resynchronize on the alternation of light and dark, returning us to the habit of being active during the day and more relaxed in the evening, even in another part of the world. **Clearly, resynchronization will not happen in 24 hours, but will take from a minimum of 2-3 days to a maximum of 14-15 days.** These particular studies are very important in the field of sports: especially if intercontinental travel is involved.
Listen to the «alarm bells» that the body uses to alert you when to «live better» every day. Every 25 hours our internal clock is «set.» The first sign of stress is then poor sleep. Norepinephrine «sets» our body's energy levels. Without norepinephrine in the brain, we will always feel tired. Norepinephrine acts as a chemical mediator of nerve transmission, it determines the transmission of nerve impulses from the fibers to the effector organs; it controls the tone of blood vessels, smooth muscles of the intestines, uterus, iris, spleen repletion, pancreatic production of insulin, and hepatic cleavage of glycogen into glucose. Low levels of norepinephrine are like trying to start a car with a dead battery. Dopamine is important for the production of endorphins, substances that among other things regulate the sense of pain and pleasure.
Stress has immunosuppressive action, through the production of norepinephrine and cortisol by the adrenal glands. In fact, stress is considered the body's «nonspecific biological response» to any environmental demand, and stressors are the various types of stimuli or agents that elicit this reaction. The nonspecific biological response, also called the general adaptation syndrome, consists of three distinct phases.
The action of **cortisol**, a hormone released by the adrenal glands during periods of alarm, influences the metabolism of sugars, proteins, and fats by increasing the body's available energy and high anti-inflammatory and antiallergic potential, and by boosting the body's defenses; however, the long-term effect is the lowering of immune defenses. Cortisol is particularly active in carbohydrate metabolism, intervenes in the sleep-wake rhythm (it is greatest during daylight hours). Increased glucocorticoids have toxic action on neurological processes. The organism declines in advance of the genetic blueprint for which it was conceived and made.
In chronic stress, the adaptive hormonal response is also chronic, leading to fatigue and general weakening. Diseases easily arise; the processes of tissue growth, turnover and repair are delayed. Stress can cause an in-

crease in the level of androgen hormones, exacerbating hair loss. This is particularly evident in women, where the level of androgens produced by the adrenal gland increases. In fact, under stress, for example, acne increases and women may miss some periods.

Very important in this paradigm is chronic stress, which, by causing hormonal changes, can be very negative.

- At the cardiac level, the following problems can be determined: tachycardia, irregular heartbeat (extrasystole), pain in the center of the chest, hypertension (although it is probably determined by heredity, diet, lifestyle habits, etc.), heart attack.
- At the lung level: bronchial asthma (asthmatic crisis triggered and maintained by anxiety), hyperventilation (rapid and shallow breathing).
- At the gastrointestinal level: irritable bowel (diarrhea, constipation, pain), dyspepsia (feeling full after a meal, acidity, belching, pain), gastroduodenal ulcer (increased acid secretion), Crohn's disease.
- At the endocrine level, stress affects the activity of peripheral endocrine glands, so adrenal glands, pancreas, kidneys, thyroid... There are some studies that hypothesize the onset of diabetes.
- At the urogenital level: premature ejaculation (in chronic anxiety), decreased desire (in depression).
- At the skin level: hyperhidrosis (excessive sweating, usually on the palm of the hand or the soles of the feet), itching, trichotillomania (the person pulls out hair, often eyelashes).

Work can be the cause of a variety of stressful situations. Even more serious is stress caused by lack of work (unemployment).

THE SYMPTOMS OF STRESS

Frequent feeling of general fatigue, accelerated heart rate, difficulty in concentration, panic attacks, crying fits, depression, anxiety attacks, sleep disturbances, muscle pain, stomach ulcer, diarrhea, stomach cramps, colitis, thyroid malfunction, high blood pressure, ease of having illnesses, inability to express oneself and find a familiar word, feeling of boredom toward any situation, frequent need to urinate, change of voice, hyperactivity, mental confusion, irritability.

Stress remedies

We talk about **managing stress, not eliminating it completely**, precisely because stress is a feature of life. One can act by intervening directly on the stressful stimuli, by changing the thoughts generated by the stressful event, through psychotropic drugs (useful in cases of acute suffering) or through relaxation techniques. The first thing to do is to try to restore the internal clock to normal levels. This process can take three weeks.

What to do?

Do not put yourself in stressful conditions, even light ones. Limit stressful situations, never losing sight of one's own well-being, one's own will. Do not bend to frustrating situations and minimize giving up. Begin to say no both to those who ask too much and more simply when one does not feel like doing something. Instead of reasoning on the basis of «why not?», begin to ask «why yes?» Always try to choose independently, without being influenced by external pressures: you will have fewer regrets, grudges and thus less stress. Devote yourself as soon as you can to something you really enjoy and enjoy, without feeling guilty about it: time spent better is just that, which allows you to regenerate yourself psychologically. Every now and then take a break and act «slowly,» savoring for example a food, looking around while walking, etc.
Evaluate each situation according to what it is, not according to what will be next. If, for example, one is on vacation, it is better to enjoy the vacation to the fullest than to become bitter thinking that perhaps it was better to do something else in the meantime. Move or skip a particular job or commitment. Avoid such thoughts as, «I must be perfect in any situation,» «I cannot refuse others' demands.» Instead, make thoughts like, «I will do this one step at a time,» «it will be okay,» «relax, keep calm,» «I have seen worse things than this,» «I can undo the worry now.»

Remember: any change is stress.

Try not to have a profligate life.

Exercise three times a week, 20 minutes to 2 hours: it will increase the production of certain positive substances.

Avoid the use of sedatives and tranquilizers: they slow the return to proper production of substances such as serotonin, norepinephrine and dopamine. If you already use such substances, you will need to stop taking them gradually and in any case under the supervision of your doctor.

Chapter 46
OB Time Machine: wellness genetics to get healthy again

«Attach your wagon to a star.»
Ralph Waldo Emerson

The aim of this Orthomolecular Biohacking manual is to provide you with the tools you need to face **the most important confrontation of your life: staying or becoming healthy again, slowing down aging, staying young as long as possible, or reaching a previously unexplored level of well-being. Bring dignity to life by achieving that added value of quality that will make us Really feel and be younger**.
Some might argue that the secret to staying young is kept within our genes, so why get so worked up, run, jump, eat well, eat better, take supplements, vitamins, amino acids, minerals - so much so that the usual relentless and cynical genetics makes the difference.

The theory of natural selection proposed by Sir Charles Darwin in 1859 predicted that it is the environment itself that selects species, facilitating the one with characteristics most compatible with the living environment. It also predicts that the driving force behind the evolution of species is the individual variability of living things that, while belonging to the same species are similar but not the same, differing widely on the basis of well-defined morphological, physiological and behavioral characteristics. As Hippocrates of Coo, the father of medicine, had already masterfully anticipated well over 2400 years ago in his De Aeribus ("The Treatise of Lands and Places"), the environment influences humans and vice versa. Depending on the environment in which one lives, some features benefit, some hinder, while others leave man's vital activity indifferent.

Genetically better-equipped individuals in an environment that is better suited to them will have an easy time. The fittest in nature are those who can obtain food more easily and mate more quickly and efficiently (i.e., procreate) than others of the same species who do not exhibit these characteristics.

Individuals with the characteristics least suited to the environmental situation will have difficulties in performing basic life functions, and many of them will fail to make it to mating, thus failing to pass on their genetic heritage to subsequent generations.

With the passage of time, generations will progressively adapt through the selection of good genes and the disappearance of unnecessary or harmful ones. The species will progressively evolve by retaining those characteristics that make it best adapted to the environment and eliminating all those that are obstacles to life. It will arrive at a situation of equilibrium between environment and population that will persist until an environmental change triggers a new evolutionary phenomenon in the species. This evolutionary phenomenon you are able to determine now, right now, by applying this OB approach. In percentage terms, the genetic responsibility toward aging can be quantified as about 60 percent, while the remaining 40 percent would be related to other factors, among which environmental influence seems to act decisively. According to the principle of survival of the fittest in the biology of the species, there seems to be no place for «weak» and «vulnerable» individuals: this is why certain genes are in charge of regulating apoptosis (cell «suicide»). Manipulation of these genes has made it possible experimentally to extend the lives of mice by 30 percent.

TELOMERES AND IMMORTALITY

Telomeres are portions of DNA located at the end of each chromosome. Their job is to protect the chromosomes during cell division; this task wears them down, and each time the cell divides, they shorten. At some point their length is no longer able to protect the cell, which reproduces incorrectly, generating aging.

What is the limitation of the telomere theory? The fact that telomeres may not be the real bottleneck of the aging process; in other words, even with telomeres of infinite length, other factors could intervene that would drastically reduce longevity.
Have cancer cells already discovered the secret of immortality? It would seem so, as scientific studies would have shown how, probably because of the enzyme telomerase, these cells are able to free themselves from the cellular accounting of the passing of time.
Telomerase is an enzyme that would repair telomeres, preventing their progressive wear and tear that results in chromosome shortening. The telomere is a kind of cap that lines the end of the chromosome. Scientists at the University of Texas, led by J.W. Shay, have acted on the telomerase enzyme, succeeding in reducing the progression of aging, but to sing definitive victory for genetics we still have a long time to wait, which is why it is advisable to start now to take care of «one's own immortality,» becoming aware of the importance of this 3-week wellness program... extendable if desired to definitely much, but much longer times and, why not, for a lifetime. It is up to you, dear readers, to decide the time frame. For the modalities needless to say, read on. By reading you increase your knowledge and only those who are in the know are able to decide and only those who decide are free.

OBESITY DEREGULATES HUMAN THE GENETIC CODE

«Obesity deregulates the genetic code while properly programmed physical activity will help you resynchronize it through proper lifestyle and healthier eating.»
A.P.

Americans Andrew Z. Fire and Craig C. Mello, recipients of the 2006 Nobel Prize in Medicine, are two molecular biologists. Both are «under 50»: 47 years old the former and 46 the latter. The two Nobel laureates have identified a «key» mechanism for exchanging genetic information: microswitches, i.e., interfering RNAs, that can silence a gene. Our genome «works» by sending instructions for protein production from the DNA in the cell nucleus to the factory in the cytoplasm. This information is transmitted by messenger RNA.
The discovery that earned the two scientists recognition, published in 1998, is precisely interfering RNA, the mechanism by which the destroy

messenger RNA from a single gene. Inside the cell, through a series of steps, a «biochemical machine» is put into operation that degrades messenger RNA molecules. In this way, the corresponding gene is turned off and the encoded protein is not produced.
This mechanism occurs in humans, animals, and plants and is vital for the regulation of gene expression, the body's defense against viral infection, and the control of genes that move «haphazardly» and can cause damage if they are in the wrong place.
It is then widely used in basic science to study gene function and may contribute to the development of new therapies against widespread diseases. Fire and Mello studied how gene expression is regulated in Caenorhabditis elegans, a nematode widely used in research. They tested their starting hypothesis by injecting double-helix RNA molecules that contained the genetic codes for several proteins in the worm in question. The effect was the same in each experiment: the gene with the code corresponding to that of the injected RNA molecules was silenced.
The results were published in Nature in February 1998, revealing a natural mechanism for controlling genetic information and opening a promising new line of research. In case of infection, for example, thanks to this mechanism, **viral RNA is degraded and the cell survives**, especially in less-developed organisms, which lack an efficient immune system, aging and longevity are not exempt, as they too are affected by gender inequalities. In fact, a new international study, conducted on data from Organization for Economic Cooperation and Development (OECD) countries, **has found that there are marked differences between men and women in both life expectancy and the way they experience old age, with important implications for a country's ability to support its elderly population.** Although, in fact, women live longer than men, they are at greater risk of developing chronic diseases, which dramatically affect their health and quality of life, as well as spending more years alone and with lower incomes. A gender gap, that of aging, intersects medicine with economic, social and cultural factors.

WHY WOMEN LIVE LONGER THAN MEN, BUT AGE WORSE

«Women eat less and therefore live longer, and it is not at all true that married men live longer. It just seems to them that life is longer.»
My Uncle Henry. Great Mentor and Friend

Worldwide, women live longer than men. The phenomenon emerged in the last years of the nineteenth century and is mainly due to gender differences in cardiovascular mortality. This is revealed in a study by researchers at Southern California University, led by Eileen M. Crimmins, who signed a paper in the Proceedings of the National Academy of Sciences. older women, while living longer than men, are more prone to chronic disease and disability.

> Although we are programmed to live to over 120 years old, we manage to use our bodies so poorly that we live much less and in often exceedingly poor conditions.

Lifestyle is everything, but often it does not take a lifetime to learn it, and perhaps just when we are about to brush up against its true meaning-that's when the hourglass of life is almost empty. Women generally have much more awareness than men, and not surprisingly they outlive males. Among the causes of early mortality, cancers play a predominant though lesser role than causes of mortality induced by cardio cerebrovascular disease.

KITCHEN OB TIPS: TELL ME HOW YOU COOK AND I'LL TELL YOU HOW YOU ARE

«To do easily what others find difficult is talent. Doing what is impossible to talent is the genius of Heinz Beck: a scientist in the kitchen.»
AP

This I learned from my friend Heinz Beck: cooking methods can make a difference all right! The way in which foods are cooked is also important. Just one example: frying potatoes with good olive oil means bringing to a very high temperature a vegetable that does not have with it any fat capable of turning into dangerous molecules. If, on the other hand, we fry eggs, fish or meat, we are bringing to very high temperatures foods rich in fats that, by hydrogenating, can become dangerous molecules. We therefore use light cooking methods.

Best cooking methods:
Gastrovac appliance (according to Heinz Beck)
steaming
boiling
stewing
baking
cooking with microwave.

Worse cooking methods:
Frying: releases acrolein;
cooking barbecuing (free benzopyrene, a highly carcinogenic molecule);
Pressure cooker: the high temperature to which the food is subjected destroys vitamin C.

BEWARE THE AGES: GENETIC RECOMBINATION OF FOODS AND DISEASES

The helm of the ship is now in the hands of the ship's Chef, and the words broadcasting from the captain's megaphone are no longer about the course ephemeris, but about what will be eaten tomorrow.
Remembering my patient and friend, the great and unforgettable Gualtiero Marchesi, I am reminded of his proverbial words after a wonderful dinner, his guest at the «Marchesino» in Milan.
«Dear Prof. Thanks to you that today I am again at the stove as much as God wills... I wanted to honor our friendship with my favorite recipe that I dedicate to you with gratitude and esteem.»

Gualtiero Marchesi's recipe: Risotto, gold and saffron

Ingredients for 4 persons:
300 gr. Carnaroli rice 80 gr. butter
20 gr. grated Parmesan cheese, 50 gr. chopped onion
200 ml. dry white wine, 1 lt. light broth
5 gr. saffron stigmas, 4 sheets of edible gold

It was he who first told me about AGES in pursuit of quality, it is the cook who must teach the customer how to eat. Cooking is in itself science, it is up to the cook to make it an art. and I am counting on you!
AGES are end products of advanced glycation of proteins or lipids that bind indissolubly by caramelizing (Maillard's Reaction) the sugars during the cooking processes and become embedded in soft tissues, creating extensive damage to endothelial and to vessels, cartilage, and joint synovium.
AGES are prevalent in the diabetic vascular system and contribute to the development of atherosclerosis, but they are still the risk of a diet that uses high and prolonged temperature cooking; it is better to prefer low-temperature cooking.
«**In one day in each cell of our body, 1,000 to 1 million molecular lesions accumulate by mistake.** Fortunately, there are proteins in the body that 'patrol' the DNA looking for errors, and repair them. One of these is called SUMO (Small Ubiquitin-like Modifier) and is able to prevent cells with damaged DNA from continuing to duplicate, giving rise to tumors and metastasis by a mechanism called 'sumoylation.'» The findings promise «potential applications in therapeutics by identifying a new therapeutic target that can be used in the future to fight cancer.» «A phenomenon known as DNA 'recombination' occurs to an excessive extent in cancer cells. Basically, at the time a cell divides to give rise to two daughter cells, genes shuffle and go to form, on the DNA of the new cells, genetic combinations different from those of the parent cell.»
Recombination is a normal phenomenon, but if cells recombine too much «the result can be 'messy' DNA, with sometimes very serious consequences.» Excessive recombination, according to experimental observations, would be associated with all types of cancers. Mutations in genes linked to the SUMO protein and in enzymes involved in 'sumoylation' have been found to lead to the accumulation of «aberrant chromosomal structures,» which block the normal process of DNA replication. In many cancers, sumoylation enzymes are present at abnormal levels. But, until now, no one had looked for mutations in sumoylation genes in the tumor types themselves. I am sure that in the next few years several will be highlighted. And these mutations will be the targets against which to target specific drugs in the anticancer therapies of the future.

On the subject of recombinant action and food-induced mutagenic effects, the opinion of Umberto Veronesi, scientific director of the European Institute of Oncology and former minister of health, who states that polenta could be carcinogenic, is significant. Traditional corn, produced in our plains, is attacked by the corn borer, an insect that digs tiny caves in the kernels and cobs, promoting, especially during the hot season, the growth of Aspergillus flavus, a mold that produces aflatoxin, a very powerful carcinogen. 2005 was a very hot year, as everyone remembers, but no one threw away the corn. Instead, it was milled and given to farms.

"Aflatoxins," the scientist continues, "are mutagenic and through various passages reach the human body. Not only through polenta, but also in milk. In this regard, a few months ago [2004] 200 tons of milk was seized, which contained very high doses of aflatoxin, but no one says so. Which means that until the day before, children were happily drinking it. It is a situation before our eyes, but nobody does anything about it...".

Chapter 47
Genetic engineering and food intolerance

«I always wanted to know as much as I could about the world.»
Linus Pauling

Although the banner of population increase is often waved to justify the abnormal and pathological development of genetic engineering, according to the World Food Program of the United Nations we are currently producing more food than is needed to feed all the inhabitants of the Planet, according to adequate nutritional values. Despite this, more than one in seven people go hungry. Genetic engineering is indispensable for the progress of humanity, but it still needs to be moderated by a "super partes" (a sage and well balanced) scientific commission, unscathed by the commercial enticements induced by unscrupulous multinational corporations, that knows how to protect the rights of humanity.
Even if genetic engineering were able to deliver on its promises of high yields and disease-resistant crops for the Third World, it seems unlikely to benefit starving populations because it does not address the root causes of malnutrition. Indeed, by claiming that this complex problem can be solved by a biotechnological panacea, governments and industries are trying to cover up the mutual complicity that allows those political structures and social inequalities responsible for the food insufficiency of millions of people to continue.
For every euro the West allocates in humanitarian aid to the Third World, 3 euros are paid by the same countries for interest on their debt. The 1997 United Nations Development Report stated that «in Africa alone, the money spent on annual debt repayment could be used to save the lives of some 21 million children.» At the time of the 1984 famine in Ethiopia, canola, flax and cotton were being grown on the most fertile

farmland for export as cattle feed to the United Kingdom and other European countries.

The biotechnological revolution thus falls into the tragic groove of the so-called Green Revolution, which ruined the lives of millions of farmers in the South for the sole benefit of countries and companies that imported cheaply abundant crops that the poor could never eat. In South Korea, following developments in the Green Revolution, the number of rural households in debt rose from 76 percent in 1971 to 98 percent in 1985; in Punjab, between 1970 and 1980, these high costs led to a reduction in the number of small farms of about 25 percent. In India, the debt problem drove many farmers to suicide. The impact of the «Green Revolution» was no less severe in Africa and South America.

It is not clear how the high investments supported by the agro-bio-technology multinationals can then be transformed into generous interventions on behalf of starving and indebted populations. Rather, there is a risk that with patents on agricultural varieties, having eliminated natural biodiversity, that these economic giants will directly appropriate seeds and thus production, and thus, with frightening social control, be able to decide (by selling or not selling the seeds) who eats and under what conditions. *(W. Bello and S. Rosenfeld, Dragons in Distress; Asia's Miracle Economies in Crisis, Institute for Food and Development Policy, 1990, San Francisco, p. 86., www.ambientediritto.it/Dossier/OGM%20Greenpeace.htm).*

FOOD INTOLERANCES AND ALLERGIES. FOOD INTOLERANT OR LIFE INTOLERANT?

Food intolerance and allergy can be the consequence of an inability to «digest» a particular food; for example, lactose intolerance, which can arise as a result of specific lactase enzyme deficiency or as a consequence of psychological factors. This type of intolerance is widespread and involves most people after weaning; therefore, it will be helpful to banish milk and dairy products from the table for these 3 weeks of the program.

A Finnish paper (J. Kokkonen et al., J Pediatr Gastroenterol Nutr 2001 Feb; 32, 2: 156-61), not very recent but made relevant by the tone of the latest controversy on the subject, has shown that milk allergy does not disappear, but rather transforms, allowing sufferers to achieve partial tolerance, which avoids acute damage but instead retains the local and general inflammatory effects typical of milk protein intolerance.

Intolerances and allergies are often and erroneously used as synonymous with each other, but in clinical reality the two situations differ like day and night. Nonetheless, many medical colleagues ignore or pretend to ignore such incontrovertible scientific objectivity, diagnosing it instead as a psychosomatic disease, denoting a pathology in which the primary action of the mind creates a damaging action in the body.

The Biohacker, like a diligent administrator, knows perfectly well that before embarking on any test to study food intolerances and allergies, it is necessary to consider the rebalancing of the MICROBIOME, that sort of intestinal condominium where each person will have to pay the management expenses in a timely manner to prevent the building from falling apart (IBS, etc.). Muhammad was quite right when he claimed that there was no more difficult vessel to fill than the stomach of the human being In fact, the more you fill it, the more it expands, and the more it requires to be filled...

In intolerances, unlike allergies proper, antigen-antibody reactions do not appear, and the immune system is much less involved. In addition, the onset of symptoms is much more nuanced in time and therefore insidious, being able to occur as late as 3 to 15 hours after primary contact with the offending substance. Such symptoms can present in a protean and variable manner, sometimes manifesting as:

- Migraine or headache;
- fatigue;
- Poor digestion (constipation, constipation, diarrhea, meteorism, colitis);
- irritability, depression, decreased ability to concentrate, mood variability, hyperkinesis (in children);
- Joint pain (sciatica, scapulohumeral periarthritis, stiff neck, etc.);
- Eczema, hives, itching, dandruff in hair, etc.

In hypersensitivities, since antibodies to invading antigens are not involved, damage to white blood cells is therefore assessed, which are examined in the «in vitro» phase with cytotoxic food intolerance tests, after separation of lymphocytes.

Food allergies, and in particular immediate reaction allergies, accompany us, with symptomatic «ups and downs», usually for our entire lives. Intolerances, on the other hand, tend to decrease if we avoid the offending food for periods d 2-4 months, and we can return to eating the same food without unpleasant side effects. However, the possibility of reaction remains, and if the food is taken too frequently (e.g., daily), the intolerance is highly likely to reoccur within 4-6 weeks, often exacerbated by a fungal infection (candida albicans type, for example), viral infection, or vaccination. A few times I have found, in more than 20 years of clinical observation, that the complaints can disappear very quickly, after a period of abstinence, not to reappear even if the patient resumes previous eating habits. Once food hypersensitivities have been ascertained, strict exclusion of dangerous substances is most important, especially in the first 20 days of the diet; in fact, already after 3 weeks of exclusion of critical foods, highlighted by Black's cytotoxic test, the body is able to get rid of about 50 percent of toxic immune complexes (aggregates of antibodies and food antigens themselves), and the patient begins to improve his or her general condition significantly, regaining serenity and zest for life.

The first 3 weeks of food exclusions are characterized by a mild flare-ups of initial symptoms, caused by the massive release of toxins from the System Endothelial Reticulum (SER). The SER is a kind of immune sponge, soaked in the toxins accumulated over months or years of dietary errors. It functions like a magnetic tape on which is recorded, with extreme fidelity, every event of our existence, from the first vaccination to the last tonsillitis of our lives. Healing is contingent upon the complete cleansing of the body system, which consists of the removal of these toxins.

OB DETOX = VICARIATE TOXINS

When we are no longer able to excrete toxins, our survival is at an end. Man is a flow system that depends on substances from outside (water, food, air, etc.). Excess, deficiency, or toxicity of the same necessarily must create disturbances. The presence of toxins is followed by defensive measures, on the part of the circulatory system, called diseases. In certain situations it is appropriate to facilitate the expulsion of this unwelcome toxin baggage through the use of appropriate nosodic and/or draining therapies. The patient, made aware of this eventuality, copes admirably with even this brief interlude in the prospect of incipient ameliorative change. This transient situation, otherwise known as regressive vicariation, is to be regarded as a prodromal phase of orthomolecular healing.

As his/her health improves, the patient gains confidence and is able to cope better and better with the exclusion diet, the immune system is strengthened and the body becomes less and less susceptible, increasing the subject's quality of life.The immune response occurs through the strengthening of our body's overall defense system and is characterized by the induction of specific enzymes, especially in the liver, antibody production, neural reflexes, and mesenchymal detoxification functions (the term mesenchyme is pseudonym for endothelial reticular system).
No allergy problem can be permanently and stably resolved unless the cause of the intoxication itself is first removed. Allergies and hypersensitivities are mainly caused by the release of histamine during inflammation, which is not completely inactivated due to pharmacological repression (caused by antibiotics, sulfa drugs, bacterial endotoxins, etc.) of which the physician too often abuses!
Overt toxic reactions must also be considered in individuals who have used foods containing large amounts of «histamine,» such as:

- Swiss cheeses;
- tuna.

Only a receptive biological terrain can be invaded by germs or toxins, triggering localized or general inflammation, and often the bacterium or, as in our case, histamine, serve as a suitable biological factor, necessary as well as useful for initiating the processes that lead to the expulsion of toxins.

The high concentration of amines found in cheese (tyramine) and chocolate (phenylethylamine) can cause reactions in sensitive individuals. In contrast, toxins in mushrooms and some fish from at-risk or otherwise polluted watersheds can sometimes lead to fatal outcomes. Beans, if consumed undercooked, can induce flatulence and intestinal meteorism (excessive gas production) or diarrhea.
Eating, for example, raw rhubarb leaves in salads rather than cooked can cause episodes of «acute gastroenteritis.» Thus, other foods often found on our table that contain high percentages of fat-soluble vitamin A can become toxic if consumed in large quantities.

NUTRIGENOMICS: GENE REPAIR DAWN OF THE NEW HUMANISM

In earlier times, the physician spent a lot of time with the patient, partly because he or she had very few tools to diagnose and treat disease. Today that more diagnostic and therapeutic efficiency of medicine is available, however, it is not able to meet all individual and societal expectations in a timely manner. Running for cover, courses on the Humanism of Medicine are being planned for medical students in the university setting.

Medicine is science and art that interpenetrate in a kind of dialectic paradigm of opposites in constant flux, which gives the humanities an intrinsic cultural value aimed at producing within themselves a thought that can unify the cognitive and practical dimensions of the harmony of body and mind, a vocation that while certainly will not allow the elaboration of magic formulas of «humanistic cures,» it will allow doctors and patients to be forged in deeper ameliorative harmony.

Genomic medicine, according to William Haseltine, founder of Human Genome Science, a regenerative medicine society, **is concerned with the proper therapeutic use of genes aimed at repairing the damage inflicted on the human body by disease and time in order to regenerate it.** However, US pediatrician and geneticist Barton Childs argues in a recent book (Genetic Medicine. A Logic of Disease, The Johns Hopkins University Press, Baltimore, 1999), that developments in genomic medicine are perhaps creating the conditions for rethinking medicine beginning with its foundations.

Rethinking medicine by considering disease as the expression of an individual limitation of adaptive capacity in relation to the environment, due to some variation at the level of the genes that control individual steps of a complex symphonic variety such as that of life. Genes, in this perspective, are the product of the evolutionary phylogeny of the species, a kind of fuse that can protect the DNA (code of life) from environmental short-circuits. Genes' prerogative function is to appropriately modulate the current flow of information reaching cells, tissues, organs that might otherwise interfere with the fine balance of life (homeostasis).

Bad lifestyle habits, pollution, transgenic foods, pesticides, fertilizers, etc. are just some of the stressors to which the body is constantly undergoing, and inducing hopefully ameliorative adaptive phenomena, mediated by the genes themselves.

P53, the guardian of the Genome (tumor suppressor protein 53) is not the pseudonym of a Masonic lodge but is the abbreviation of a gene, TP 53, which regulates the cell cycle and is capable of suppressing the development of tu-

mors even before they can be photographed by a CT scan, PET scan, MRI, etc. Such a marvelous and almost tireless system is active 24 h/day and woe if it stops... It would be like being in the middle of Antarctica with a snowmobile without gasoline... Or in a more prosaic and parochial way, to start cheering "Forza Lazio" in the "south curve" at the Stadio Olimpico while the derby is being played... The Genome Keeper abandons the workplace when he is subdued by excessive stress, summarized in a bad lifestyle with ex-cessive oxidation-reduction («rusting») of his cellular terrain.
As the French hydrologist Louis Claude Vincenti argued, «the soil and all the germ nothing.» Therefore, we must have not good, but excellent care in a preventive sense of our lifestyles, otherwise we cannot then complain about the latency of P53...
By placing the origin of diseases in a perspective that is simultaneously functional (biochemical), genetic, and evolutionary, the result is that each patient is a unique manifestation of disease and not its opposite, that is, a typical case of disease with equally unique treatment needs. Since genetic vulnerabilities create inconsistencies with particular aspects of the environment, including social organization and culture, it follows that as much effort should be directed in the search for preventive environmental conditions as in the search for treatments.

Genomic medicine will tend to be the medicine of the person: unique and individual, and will involve not only individuals already suffering from dis-ease, but evidently apparently healthy individuals who carry some genetic susceptibility to becoming ill. Genomic medicine will treat the healthy, true to the Chinese aphorism that urged to remunerate the physician only when one was healthy, ceasing to do so when disease took over, as a harbinger of an essential error in the setting of the doctor-patient relationship. The physician will be able to inform the patient extensively, even to the point of predicting whether and when he or she may suffer from a disease of greater or lesser severity during his or her future existence. **All this will necessarily impose on the health care professional a continuous and constant updating on the developments of research that is changing the taxonomy of diseases, better focusing all the more accurate and sincere communication strategies.**

The redistribution of populations on the basis of genetic traits is based on clear and irrefutable ethical norms that ensure the protection of the individ-ual to the end that no category is discriminated against, allowing the devel-opment of fair and supportive research to improve quality of life and health.

The frontiers of Nutrigenomics seem to be opening new vistas in cancer prevention, revisiting its absolute significance. This disease is now viewed as a chronic genome event that can be influenced, at many stages of the patient's natural history, by nutritional and metabolic factors that affect not only the prevention but also the progression and treatment of this devastating disease. The cancer phenotype is the result of the interaction of both gene and environmental influences. Most of the evidence in this area pertains to both studies performed on human populations and experiments performed on animals, which model the process of carcinogenesis. Undoubtedly, the most obvious and indisputable environmental influence is that based on diet. It has been estimated that up to 80% of breast and prostate neoplasms and one-third of all cancer diseases can be influenced by diet and associated lifestyle factors.

All categories of classical nutrients consist of the bioactive dietary residues, including carbohydrates, amino acids, fatty acids, lipids, minerals, and structural vitamins. There is, however, an extensive list of components of non-nutrient substances, especially phytochemicals (components found in plants) that may have remarkable antineoplastic and antimutagenic activity (D.M. Harris and V.L.W. Go, «How dietary components protect from cancer»; in Nutrition and Cancer Prevention, edited by A.B. Awad and P.G. Bradford, Marcel Dekker, New York, 2005, pp. 27-58).

More than 25,000 different chemical residues are found in fruits and vegetables and other plants consumed by humans. Included in these category codes are substances such as: **carotenoids, flavonoids, organosulfates, isothiocyanates, indoles, monoterpenes, phenolic acids, and chlorophyll** (C.D. Davis and J. Milner, «Frontiers in nutrigenomics, proteomics, metabolomics and cancer prevention,» Mutation Research, July 13, 2004, 551 (1-2): 51-64). Most of these nutrients can influence gene expression, and dietary habits continue to emerge as significant factors capable of influencing cancer incidence and tumor behavior. According to Alan Jackson, **nutritional programming in utero has an important effect on the development of chronic diseases later in life** (A.A. Jackson, «Integrating the ideas of life course, cellular, individual and population levels in cancer causation,» The Journal of Nutrition, Dec. 2005, 135 (12 suppl.): 2927S-2933S).

It is essential to measure new biomarkers of substance-gene interaction in genotype-phenotype continuity at different stages of the life cycle and to identify responders and non-responders to a particular diet. Thus, nutritional genomics holds broad potential in the prevention of chronic-degenerative diseases and provides a new frontier, that of challenging the establishment of an individualized health program (J.B. German, D.E Bauman, D.G. Burrin, et al. «Metabolomics in the opening decade of the 21st century: building the roads to individualized health,» J Nutr., Oct. 2004; 134 (10): 2729- 2732). With the advent of the postgenomic era, biological and medical research and clinical practice **witnessed an explosion in the strategies and goals of classical nutrition**, now positioned on Ground Evidence Medicine [evidence-based medicine] using evidence from Nutrigenomics (V.L. Go, D.A. Wong, Y. Wang et al., «Diet and cancer prevention: evidence-based medicine to genomic medicine,» J Nutr., Dec. 2004; 134 (12 suppl.): 3513S-3516S).

To achieve this goal requires the input of bioinformatics. To process the information stored in a database in such a way that it can only meet the needs of science once coordinated with other clinical variables such as: family and personal history, physical examinations, and functional and laboratory information, and image formation of the individual. This is the great challenge before us, but it is also a great opportunity in the dawn of nutritional genomics.

Chapter 48

Genetic profiling: What if the geniuses were thinking?

«Two things fill the soul with ever new and growing admiration and veneration... The saddled sky above me and the moral law within my DNA.»
Emmanuel Kant modified by A.P.

This OB manual will not change your genetics, rest assured, but it will help you express the potential in them.

> Genes are not inescapable judges but extremely delicate and attuned environmental reactors, endowed with a reactive-adaptive capacity that represents a form of intelligence, understood as the innate set of functions aimed at learning and solving problems, such as environmental pollution, and in a sense understanding the ideas and language of the world around us.

Genes contain information that can help assess risk for certain diseases and achieve optimal health status and performance levels. With the completion of this first phase of the Human Genome Project, scientists now hold the cards to examine more than 40,000 human genes. Today, more than 10,000 single nucleotide polymorphisms (SNPs), also known as «snips,» have been identified; these are single nucleotide mutations (the building blocks of DNA) in a gene that can have a huge impact on health status. Think of DNA as a place where cells manufacture a product-in this case, proteins: a SNP corresponds to the breaking malfunction of a machine, but if one of the machines on the assembly line is malfunctioning, the final product will be defective. **A SNP produces defective proteins.** Genomic medicine can help in preventive planning and optimization by amplifying some genetic benefits. In the area of prevention, genomic medicine takes a crucial role in what concerns the predictive aspect, identifying the polymorphisms for preventive purposes, that is, by looking for those gene- tic mutations that respond to some extent to lifestyle changes including orthomolecular nutrition, supplementation (as provided in this program) or drug treatment. If a SNP of a bone formation marker (COL1A1) is found in a patient, the individual will exhibit abnormal collagen formation leading to reduced bone density and consequent increased risk of osteoporosis. This potential problem could be solved by taking higher amounts of calcium, moderate exposure to sunlight or vitamin D supplementation.

Representatives of NuGenix and sister company GeneLink (which performs the genetic testing) in the U.S. believe they are able to detect «defects» by measuring oxidative stress, bone density, obesity, immune function, cardiovascular health, vitamin metabolism, and inflammatory genes in DNA samples. In case of deficiencies, they suggest specific supplements to make up the deficiency. But is it a safe technology?

Claude Bouchard, world-renowned geneticist, obesity researcher and executive director of the Pennington Biomedical Research Center at Louisiana State University, does not believe this at all: «This is a valid theory, but premature. **The main question is knowing which SNPs to look for.** We can say that personalized nutrition systems, based on DNA, pharmacotherapy and other lifestyle components, will be sufficiently efficient to take on considerable importance in the near future.» Jim Simpkins, coauthor of the genetic profiling reports at GeneLink and chair of the Department of Pharmacology and Neuroscience at the University of North Texas Health Science Center, is more optimistic: «The technology around SNPs is at a fairly advanced level. However, we need to find out whether genetic predisposition is really linked to premature aging (and disease).» Simpkins is confident in the studies done at GeneLink on SNPs, although he does not yet have firm evidence of direct involvement of SNPs in a particular disease. The potential applications of this new technology (once perfected) are not to be underestimated. Bruce Ames, professor of biochemistry and molecular biology at the University of California, agrees with Bouchard: «Some SNPs may not be related to diet, but our knowledge is still limited.»

While acknowledging the difficulty of combining preliminary technology and individualized nutritional advice, **Ames argues that it can work in some cases, at least with regard to some diseases, including cardio-vascular disease, cancer and Alzheimer's**: "I think our article in the Journal of Clinical Nutrition was the first to provide a logical justification for the use of supplements by some individuals. We showed that supple-mentation can reduce the risk of developing certain diseases based on the study of SNPs."

GENOMIC MEDICINE: THE LONGEVITY GENE

"It is not true that we have little time. The truth is that we waste a lot of it."
Seneca

It could be an exceptional discovery made by a German researcher, Felix Knauf, announced Oct. 29, 2005, in Berlin. Knauf, who works at the prestigious Max Delbrueck research center in the German capital, has in fact deciphered the secrets of the so-called longevity gene, found in various types of animals-from insects to mammals-that enables individuals to live much longer than their peers.

Central to life extension is a protein developed from the mutant gene, a protein responsible for utilizing carbohydrates, fat and other suitable substrates to produce energy. Knauf, studying fruit flies, has highlighted the longevity gene, a kind of protein that imposes a series of dietary restrictions on the body by reducing the absorption of food and therefore calories: this is enough, in the case of the fruit fly, even to double its life span; in the case of mammals, perhaps a little less but certainly to a significant degree. We are at the dawn of genetic research, such a complex and broad field with still poorly delineated boundaries; however, the discovery of the functioning of the longevity gene opens up new scenarios, should they also be applicable to the human model.

It is plausible to hypothesize a therapeutic and pharmacological breakthrough in the future by using the mutant gene to stimulate the production of this protein, enabling even those who are not fortunate enough to possess this fully functioning longevity gene or who do not possess it at all to curb calorie absorption by prolonging life. It will certainly take years of research. In the meantime, while genes and proteins are at work, instead of waiting, better to start now to get into the heart of the wellness project, the cornerstone of this book.

Chapter 49

Anti-aging keys: the seven anti-aging keys

«Everything belongs to the gods; the wise are friends of the gods; the goods of friends are common. Therefore the wise possess all things.»

Diogenes the Cynic

As evidenced by several researches conducted on centenarians on the island of Okinawa, Japan, and in some villages of Gennargentu, Sardinia, genes seem in part to determine the original imprint of a more or less lenghty life, and on which it is not yet possible to intervene. Much, however, can already be done on good habits. One can use this OB handbook as a starting point. Planned movement, diet and supplementation of amino acids, vitamins, minerals and herbal medicines, plenty of low-cluster water, and above all, no smoking. A modest and balanced diet, rich in vegetables, without overdoing fruit (watch out for kiwis), pre and probiotics and few grains, preferably whole grains, if tolerated. Protein in the right amount without excess or deficiency. All seasoned with EVO (extra virgin olive oil, but no bread and pasta, which may be eaten only exceptionally, basically the Mediterranean food model, but with some modifications.

As several studies have shown, for example the one published in the New England Journal of Medicine, extra virgin olive oil contains not only a large amount of monounsaturated fatty acids, but also polyphenolic compounds capable of both counteracting the oxidation of biological macromolecules such as DNA, proteins and lipids, as well as boosting the body's endogenous cellular antioxidant defenses, which is equivalent to saying that it would be enough to introduce at least 25 ml of extra virgin olive oil into the diet daily to benefit from a very powerful anti-aging OB strategy. To rebalance the intestinal asset, one needs to pay special attention to the diet.

It is definitely useless, or at least chronologically less effective, to administer supplements without changing lifestyle habits and especially without first performing a detoxification procedure (OB DETOX). Aging alters not only organs and tissues but also the microbiota, which is the community of microbes living inside the body and on its surface. Some changes in this microbial population depend on lifestyle; others, however, are a consequence of the passage of years. Acting on them can help you age while maintaining good health.

A proper Orthomolecular Biohacking program must aim first and foremost at physiological rebalancing, which relies on a range of formulas, means and remedies, often of natural origin or from Orthomolecular Medicine, that target the seven main targets of aging:

skin (photoaging)

appetite

memory

mood

sleep

sex hormones

muscles.

These are the keys or, rather, the organs and functions most affected by advancing years, complicit in the progressive, lower production of hormones and neurotransmitters.

Analysis of the microbiome makes it possible to identify any alterations in the microbiota by studying its genes and, consequently, to identify the most appropriate strategies to promote good health by acting on the detected imbalances.

A program based Orthomolecular Biohacking on endo- modulation, or the targeted administration of cocktails of nutrients-vitamins, amino acids, minerals-hormone and neurotransmitter precursors useful for targeting the targets of so-called aging.

Key 1: Skin and tan.

Of all the targets of aging, certainly the skin is the most conspicuous. After the age of 50, the skin of women especially (but also men) changes in relation to intrinsic, extrinsic, hormonal, and physical factors. Intrinsic factors are responsible for genetically programmed aging and result in

progressively pale, thin, hypoelastic skin and wrinkles. In particular, menopause affects women. Extrinsic factors, in addition to lifestyles, include the strong impact on the skin of photoaging, i.e., aggressions from the external environment, such as the sun, guilty not only of ultraviolet rays, but also of incorrect exposure, which can induce the onset of wrinkles, solar keratosis, skin dyschromia (spots), a situation that predisposes to inflammatory and degenerative type reactions induced by ultraviolet radiation, especially following occasional and sudden exposure, as happens especially in winter following trips to the tropics or weekends in the mountains at high altitude.
Deferring to specialist countermeasures, skin-specific anti-aging treatments today range from the appropriate introduction of nutrients (antioxidants) to hormonal drugs, via more or less deep topical interventions, such as peels, fillers, lasers, and facelifts. For all, of course, it is imperative to hydrate by remineralizing the skin, both during exposure and upon return, for 4-8 weeks, perhaps taking some homeo- phytotherapeutic remedies to help decongest the skin from the effects of the sun, such as Hamamelis, Fucus vesiculosus, Laminaria, etc. If there is evidence of previous sun damage to the skin, homeopathic plant DNA and RNAs, which have a repairing action, may also help.

Key 2: Appetite.

Among the first organs to age are the stomach and intestines; it is well known that overeating promotes greater production of free radicals, which, together with a weakened intestinal immune system, increases the risk of also developing forms of cancer. In addition, as is well known, overeating predisposes one to obesity and metabolic syndrome, which in turn open up problems of various kinds and severity, such as diabetes. It is most important to increase physical activity and always diet under medical supervision, especially in the presence of excess visceral fat at risk. When appetite presses and takes on a compulsive connotation, it is important to combine diet and psychotherapy, to resolve any emotional disturbances.
On the other hand, for those who want to curb an appetite that is just a little more aggressively than usual, orthomolecular therapy is undoubtedly the first choice through the administration of tryptophan and phenylalanine supplements, precursors of serotonin and cholecystokinin, respectively, which are involved in the mechanism of satiety.
To prevent hunger attacks, the rule of eating every 60-90 minutes, perhaps

a simple anti-hypoglycemia snack typical of mid-morning and afternoon, also applies. It is useless to follow drastic and monotonous diets that expose one to dangerous relapses (yo-yo syndrome) that damage the connective tissues that like a balloon continuously inflate and deflate. In these cases, it is useful to stimulate in acupuncture the so-called centers of gratification and pleasure that, when activated (even a simple but vigorous digital massage is enough), stimulate the release of serotonin in the brain, such as point 8 of the gallbladder (GB8), which is located on the temple, above the ear. Stimulate this point four times a day at regular intervals throughout the day for at least one continuous minute following clockwise with your fingertip, perhaps using your fingernail, almost as if it were a needle, until you evoke an almost intolerable discomfort (not pain). Continue undeterred for at least 10 days and you will be surprised at the effects: try it to believe!

Key 3: Memory.

It is from the age of 40 that the cerebral cortex begins to age, losing a significant number of neurons (about 40,000 per day), decreasing the synthesis of neurotransmitters and the number and sensitivity of receptors. For this reason, problems such as memory loss, difficulty in concentration, mood alterations and sleep-wake rhythm disturbances become more pronounced as the years go by.

If the mnemonic damage is extensive, it will be necessary under medical supervision to investigate possible degenerative diseases, and once these risks have been ruled out, a specific O.B. strategy can be set up. It is worthwhile in this regard to consult the site of Gianni Golfera (www.gigotec.com), who is at the forefront of the art of memory, in which he has developed teaching techniques that are quick to learn and efficacious in courses lasting as little as a weekend.

Keys 4-5: mood and sleep-wake rhythm disorders.

Complex and significant, especially from old age onward, are the psychic and behavioral changes, with mild and moderate depressive streaks, mood swings, and sleep disturbances. Situations that are established mainly due to the physiological decrease in the synthesis of neurotransmitters - serotonin, norepinephrine, dopamine, GABA - to which is added the slowdown in the production of hormones, GH (growth hormone) and melatonin included, which is known to regulate sleep-wake rhythms.

In addition to preserving the most active quality of social life possible, which is an excellent antidote to depression related to aging-induced isolation, this path taken at a slower pace allows for obtain splendid results, it being understood that obviously the most challenging cases will have to be treated in any case with specific medical interventions. In less pronounced forms, and always under medical supervision, some phytotherapeutic remedies may be useful, such as Hypericum, with its well-known antidepressant properties. Bach flowers also offer help: Wild Rose for apathy, Willow if one tends to blame others, Chicory for feelings of emotional exclusion. Among the California flowers, Chrysanthemum is the most specific for those who do not psychologically accept entering old age. For insomnia: in addition to drug therapies, phototherapy and, especially for psychophysiological insomnia, cognitive-behavioral interventions are useful.

Keys 6-7: alteration and decrease in sex hormones and muscles (sarcopenia).

With advancing years, the production of sex hormones gradually slows, a process that in women culminates in menopause. In both sexes, testosterone availability also decreases, with repercussions mainly on sex life (decreased desire), but also on other organs. For example, on the brain, where it promotes reduced concentration, depression and insomnia. Lower testosterone also affects the muscles, which lose volume and facilitate fatigue. This program is useful to counteract altered sex hormones and decreased libido jointly with arginine and ornithine, precursors of growth hormone.

It goes without saying that for libido, an excellent workout always remains the maintenance of sexual activity as well as good muscular level is maintained over the years with the constant movement provided by the program, adjusted to the health conditions that involves the consensual practice of a gentle discipline, such as Qi Gong and Tai Chi Chuan. For decreased libido, various remedies such as those from traditional Chinese pharmacology can also help.

Ginseng decoction and Angelica, among others, are used for their action on sex hormones and mood. Also indicated in women is the Liu Wei Di Huang Wan complex formula, based mainly on a plant, Rehmanniaglutinosa, which also combats menopausal disorders. All remedies, in each case, are to be taken under strict medical supervision.

Chapter 50

Study of the function of HGH

(Growth and wellness hormone and peptides)

«A tree whose trunk can barely be embraced springs from a tiny sprout. A tower nine stories high begins with a mound of earth. A long journey of a thousand miles begins with moving a foot.»

Lao Tse

The progressive aging of the population has made Italy one of the countries with the highest percentage of elderly individuals, placing increasing emphasis on the social and health problems associated with these age groups. Worldwide, life expectancy is currently, on average, over 71 years for men and about 76 years for women, and this, together with the reduction in fertility, has brought the percentage of over-65s to 16 percent, while young people under 15 are about 15 percent.
Moreover, demographic data suggest that this is also a very complex phenomenon from a territorial point of view, with profound diversity. Such profound changes in the structure of the population will lead to enormous problems in the adjustment of social and health care facilities, which only a more complete understanding of the aging processes, the morbid forms that accompany it, and the characteristics of aging in good health will enable. O.B. aims to improve across the board the quality of life of individuals of all age groups. Training and Intermittent Fasting, supported by the proper supplementation of amino acids, minerals and vitamins, phytotherapeutics, homeopathics, etc. allow you to maximize the reparative capacity of your tissues by helping you to achieve your desired state of form. This function is regulated by and dependent on the efficiency of individual growth factors, which tend to cluster into large families of structurally and

evolutionarily similar proteins. Famous, for example, are the families of TGF-beta (transforming growth factor), BMP (bone morphogenetic protein), neurotrophins (NGF, BDNF, and NT3), FGF (fibroblast growth factor), and so on.

Other fairly well-known growth factors are:

- Cytokine (Cytobalance)
- Granulocyte-colony stimulating factor (G-CSF)
- Granulocyte-macrophage colony stimulating factor (GM-CSF)
- Nerve growth factor (NGF)
- Neurotrophins
- Platelet-derived growth factor (PDGF)
- Erythropoietin (EPO)
- Thrombopoietin (TPO)
- Myostatin (GDF-8)
- Growth Differentiation Factor-9 (GDF9)
- Basic fibroblast growth factor (bFGF or FGF2)
- Epidermal growth factor (EGF)
- Hepatocyte growth factor (HGF).

In the U.S., peptide therapy is already widespread and is partly supplanting hormone replacement therapy, or at least being used as supportive therapy in anti aging clinics. The success of this approach is that, in contrast to hormone replacement therapies, which in most cases suppress endogenous production, peptides stimulate endogenous production and thus never lead to excessively supraphysiological values.

Let us now look at some of the most widely used of these:

INSULIN GROWTH FACTOR - 1 (IGF-1)

IGF-1 is a growth factor involved in tissue regeneration (muscle, liver, bone, brain).

This growth factor is secreted on the basis of the trauma suffered in larger or smaller amounts by fibroblasts, myocytes, immune cells, neurons, cardiomyocytes, or hepatocytes following organ damage. IGF-1 tends to be hypo-expressed with advancing age, and with it individual regenerative capacity also declines.

During aging, the biochemical pathways inherent in the action of IGF- 1 after binding to its receptor are particularly altered in skeletal muscle, which exhibits a decline in protein synthesis, as well as an increase in connective tissue and triglycerides, susceptibility to atrophy, and increased apoptosis. Conversely, overexpression or otherwise increased IGF-1 levels constitutes a protective action against sarcopenia.

Immunodeficiency, oxidative stress, fibrosis, visceral adiposity, heart failure, and neurodegeneration are other conditions inversely related to serum IGF-1 levels.

DES-IGF1 is an analogue of IGF-1 with the absence of the last 3 amino acids in the N-terminal tail; this modification makes it capable of both a higher affinity for its receptor and a longer half-life, as it resists binding to IGF-binding proteins, the proteins responsible for limiting its intracellular bioavailability.

MECCHANO GROW FACTOR WITH GLYCOL POLYETHYLENES (MGF)

MGF is a growth factor produced by muscle and liver cells subsequent to mechanical stress or stimulation with growth hormone (GH).

In contrast to IGF-1 (insulin-like growth factor 1), MGF is produced exclusively by skeletal muscle and has as its main role both the activation of satellite cells, i.e., quiescent cells located in the connective tissue that surrounds individual muscle fibers (endomysium), and the proliferation of myoblasts derived from their activation.

MGF turns out to be an essential hormone for the initiation of the myocyte regeneration process especially after intense exercise or accidental muscle damage.

In the aging process where levels of somatotropic hormones (GH, MGF, IGF) tend to drop precipitously, it has been found that GH supplementation after a training stimulus preferentially increases MGF levels over levels of the other hormones involved in the process of muscle regeneration.

Especially under conditions of muscle damage, the use of MGF combined with balanced doses of IGF-1 makes sense to speed regeneration of tissues previously stressed by intense training.

Furthermore, the decline in the synthesis of these growth factors gives way to inflammatory conditions that gradually lead to muscle tissue whose inefficiency is due to the presence of abundant connective tissue directly related to insulin resistance, inflammation, and aging.

Prevention of myocardial aging and neuroprotection are other contexts where FGM can be used for preventive purposes.

GHRP-6

Grow hormone releasing peptide-6 (GHRP6) is a stimulant of GH secretion first described in 1984 by Bowers et al.

Compared with the other GHRPs (MK-677 and GHRP2), GHRP6 was the first effective drug to raise GH levels through stimulation of ghrelin receptors (GHSR1a), an oestrous hormone produced by the stomach under fasting conditions.

The use of GHRP is recommended in those conditions where appetite stimulation, muscle regeneration, immune prevention, and neuro senescence are sought.

Both ghrelin and GH are very important peptides for maintaining immune well-being as immune cells themselves produce GH in order to differentiate, proliferate, synthesize antibodies, synthesize major histocompatibility complexes, including at the nerve level through increased proliferation of microglia, which serve as an endogenous pool of neurotrophic molecules such as IGF-1, and by promoting autophagy and consequent decreased neuroinflammation.

GHRP-2 (PRALMORELIN, KP-102)

Grow hormone releasing peptide - 2 (GHRP2) is a stimulant of GH secretion first unveiled in 1993 by Dr. Cyril Y Bowers.

Compared with GHRP6, GHRP2 results in greater stimulation of GH secretion and less appetite sensation. In circumstances where anti-aging therapy aims at improving body mass index (BMI) and on normalizing physiological GH levels, GHRP-2 is a better choice than its predecessor GHRP-6. Like GHRP- 6, GHRP-2 belongs to a class of drugs that mimic the functions of ghrelin, an endogenous peptide produced by the stomach during periods of fasting.

In addition to their recognized effects on body composition and hunger, ghrelin agonists such as GHRPs are still being tested for their potential positive effects on sleep, modulation of systemic and brain inflammation and on improving insulin sensitivity in the long term.

After a series of clinical trials, GHRP-2 was tried in 2005 in Japan as a drug to treat growth hormone deficiency states and only later in 2012 began to be used in the U.S. through Sella Pharmaceuticals where it is still used by clinics specializing on hormone replacement and anti-aging therapies.

FRAGMENT - 176-191

Fragment is a fragment of human growth hormone (hGH); numbers 176-191 indicate that the peptide contains exclusively the last 16 carboxy-terminal amino acids of the GH molecule.

Although derived directly from GH, the effects of Fragment are exclusively lipolytic and can be used for anti-aging purposes because, as age progresses, progressive metabolic slowdown, muscle catabolism, and a state of low grade inflammation prevent the body from utilizing the fat reserves in adipose tissue to the fullest as an energy substrate.
The mechanism underlying the lipolytic action of this compound is given by the activation of PKC resulting in phosphorylation and activation of HSL (hormone-sensitive lipase), an enzyme responsible for the release of triglycerides from adipose tissue.
Furthermore, it has been seen that Fragment, through the inhibition of Acetyl coa carboxylase, prevents the establishment of lipogenesis, or the formation of new adipose tissue.
A hepatoprotectant is recommended during its use in order to limit oxidative stress resulting from the release of toxic substances previously contained in the patient's adipose tissue.
Physical activity should always be performed in order to improve the oxidation of released fatty acids.

PT-141 (BREMELANOTIDE) AND MELANOTAN II

Melanotan II, or Melanotan Peptide, is a synthetic variant of a naturally occurring peptide hormone, alpha-melanocyte stimulating hormone or MSH that is responsible for melanogenesis (a process that causes skin pigmentation) in the body.
Synthetic peptide hormone manufactured and injectable is commonly used to improve sexual stamina and darken skin pigment with protective effect against sunburn from sun exposure. Melanotan II was initially developed in the 1990s at the University of Arizona led by a well-known dermatologist, Norman Levine. During testing, one of the people who had taken the drug reported to Levine that he was experiencing spontaneous erections as a result of it. Bremelanotide (derived from Melanotan II) is most potent as an inducer of sexual arousal and is a nonspecific melanocortin receptor agonist.
These receptors can be found in 5 different isoforms with function strictly dependent on their location. Bremelanotide acts on MT3 and MT4 receptors, which mainly affect appetite (modulation of neuropeptide Y), libido (through increasing oxytocin), anxiety (through increasing BDNF (brain derived growth factor), an important growth factor for neurogenesis).
Dosage should always be modulated based on side effects such as migraine

and nausea, which may occur due to the effects of these substances on blood pressure modulation.
The effects of melanocortin derivatives are not limited to libido, modulation of anxiety, and appetite, but have an immunomodulatory role that can be useful in both immunodeficiency and autoimmune skin diseases (vitiligo, psoriasis).

THYMOSIN ALPHA 1

Thymosin alpha 1 (Ta1) is a natural substance produced by the thymus gland and has been known for many years.
It is a peptide, that is, a very short protein consisting of 28 amino acids, which can also be produced by synthesis.
Its function is anti-inflammatory as well as to regulate certain immune processes.
As an immunomodulator it has long been used in viral infections, immunodeficiencies, some cancers, and AIDS.
In Italy, the indication recommended by the Ministry of Health is only as an adjunct to influenza vaccination in immunocompromised individuals.
Thymosins are biologically active and physiologically present substances in the human body that can play a regulatory function in many essential biological processes, for the proper functioning of the immune system and regenerative processes of the damaged tissues from ischemic events such as myocardial infarction and ulcers from vascular insufficiency but also from trauma and injury.

THYMOSIN BETA 4

The beneficial clinical effects of Thymosin alpha 1 result from activation of the TLR 9 receptor in dendritic cells and other cells of the immune system, such as macrophages and Natural Killer cells, with viral replication inhibition effects.
Thymosin alpha 1 has been used clinically in pilot studies for the treatment of severe acute respiratory syndrome (SARS) and other lung infections, including acute respiratory distress syndrome and chronic obstructive pulmonary disorder.
Importantly, Thymosin alpha 1 also leads to an increase in Treg lymphocytes that produce the anti-inflammatory cytokine interleukin 10, triggering an inhibitory feedback of inflammatory cytokine production, thus exerting a potent anti-inflammatory effect and attenuating the immune response and preventing cytokine storm.

Thymosin alpha 1 is currently approved in more than 37 countries for the treatment of hepatitis B and C and as an immunostimulant in numerous other diseases.
In view of a possible non-positive response to a possible vaccine for SARS-COV-2, especially in the elderly who have an impaired response, compared to the young, due to the gradual decline in Thymus function, Thymosin Alpha 1 could be considered.
Prof. Luigina Romani, at the Department of Experimental Medicine, University of Perugia, worked on Thymosin alpha 1 in 2006 with preclinical study, showing that the substance could beneficially affect chronic lung inflammation induced by infectious agents.
Other peptides worth mentioning are: TB 500 or Thymosin beta 4; BPC-157; MOTS-c; Kisspeptin-10; GHK-Cu; Epitalon; CJC-1295 and many more.

Chapter 51

Exploring the Future of Sports: The Integration of Artificial Intelligence and Sports Biohacking

«Creativity consists in imagining something that does not exist and making its existence possible.»

Brené Brown

If we look at the world of film or the world of novels related to the world of science fiction, we can already glimpse a glimmer (perhaps stereotypical in form) of what of how AI could potentially be used in our reality. If we delve, for example, into the world of video game culture (so-called videgames), we can indeed always see in the science fiction universe the various possibilities on the use of AI.
This feature of the video game (like the cinematic world, novels) highlights through sci-fi universes, various eventual applications of AI such as: technical operator, medical or armed assistance, typographical analyst, etc. and that will go on various forms help the protagonist (and the player) in the arc of his adventures. Let us remember that AI is also used in video games themselves to enhance the player's experience, adjust the difficulty according to skill level, create more realistic and responsive non-player characters, and to optimize the efficiency of gameplay.
Re-evaluating the myriad facets of sophisticated AI from science fiction, we can in a completely surprising way observe of the eventual applicative possibilities of AI extended to optimizing the professional experience of other reference figures such as the doctor, teacher, physiotherapist, sports coach, etc..
In our case and over the course of this chapter, we will see the potential for using AI intended for optimizing the biohacking experience in sports.

SPORTS AND ARTIFICIAL INTELLIGENCE: APPLICATIONS AND DEVELOPMENTS

We can observe nowadays that current technology though less «impressive» is not so far from the playful imaginary. If we look at history, digital technologies; have and are continually revolutionizing work settings in various industries, becoming an integral part of our daily lives. The applications are numerous: from voice recognition systems to route tracking applications, medicine (preventive or predictive medicine), information technology, finance (data analysis, programming) and sports. The introduction of computers has narrowed the gap between developed and developing countries by ensuring optimal and specialized use of technology. At present, artificial intelligence technology is leading humanity to enter a new era of human-machine collaboration, cross-border integration, sharing and promotion of education toward modernization, digitization, intelligent direction of continuous development, Internet of Things, big data and artificial intelligence for sports to realize a variety of possibilities. In other words, AI has proven to be a strong transformative force, not only in traditional technology-focused fields but in diverse fields (Qi et al, 2024).
But let's focus on the context of sports by first defining what AI is. According to Copeland (2023), artificial intelligence (AI) is a branch of computer science that focuses on creating intelligent machines capable of performing tasks that require human intelligence. These tasks include reasoning, meaning discovery, generalization, and learning from prior experience. Applications of AI range from advanced web search engines and recommendation systems to self-driving cars and strategic games.
The term AI was coined in 1956 and became more popular today due to advances in science and technology such as increasing data volumes and the development of algorithms and computations. In the early stages, AI research was associated with topics such as problem solving and symbolic methods. In later stages, AI developed with machine learning and today can perform processes such as language, image and data recognition, make predictions. Learning enables AI to continue to evolve. AI and machine learning are not the same thing. AI is a broad field that includes many subfields, including Machine Learning. Machine Learning is a subset of AI that is an application of AI that enables the machine or system to learn and improve automatically from experience (Kaya, 2023).
In the sports sphere, we can equally observe the same trend of 'technology integration growing in the sports sphere in all its forms by inventing serv-

ices that will optimize the experience, athletic, technical and general business. Today, advanced and scientific technologies are increasingly seen as indispensable by coaches or cutting-edge stadiums across the planet. Such a coach/machine alliance strengthens and improves sports training performance and raises the level of training globally. From a media or commercial point of view, various sports clubs can also reach more fans around the world through their promotional products and merchandising, thus earning more profits (Li, Hsieh, Fan, 2024). The Internet provides an easy access to the latest information, research, training or other sports achievements, bypassing the need to have to travel from home. Many renowned sports universities around the world make their information available to everyone through the Internet.

At present, various technical and engineering groups are incorporating AI into various scientific and technological fields, which in turn spill over into many other areas. They may relate to: improving athletes' performance and health, preparing training and diet plans, match analysis, strategy development, refereeing, player recruitment and scouting, match prediction, ticket sales, and sports journalism. According to Kaya (2023), the main benefits would include:

- ***AI-enhanced coaching:*** AI can have a significant impact on the strategic decisions coaches make before, during, and after the game. With the help of sensors and speed cameras, AI programs can calculate advanced passes, penalty shots and other relevant activities in different sports. This information will enable coaches to train players for each game and create more robust training programs for their teams.
- ***Improving player performance:*** AI can be used to improve player performance by analyzing data and providing various technical insights. Moreover, it improves the physical performance status of athletes, assess and analyze sports posture, analyze probabilistic winning rules, comfort a suitable mental state before competition, and prevent sports injuries through evaluations, rehabilitation planning (Desai, 2024), and assist staff and athlete in decision-making procedures (Liu, Hang, 2024).
- ***Improving decision-making and forecasting:*** the role of AI in decision-making and forecasting in sports is rapidly expanding and attracting increasing attention in both academia and industry. AI can also be used to analyze large datasets in sports medicine.
- ***Data analysis:*** AI can be used to analyze data obtained from games and training sessions to help coaches make more statistically successful

decisions. It identifies athletes' strengths and weaknesses, areas for improvement, advantages and disadvantages compared to their opponents.

- ***Simulation of training scenarios:*** AI can provide specific support to athletes' physical education in various ways, such as data analysis and simulation through potential training scenarios. For example, they can provide computer vision to analyze athletes' movements, highlight the use of natural language to understand athletes' speech, and use of data mining to evaluate athletes' performance.

In terms of applications, Kaya (2023) also highlights four main categories of AI applications.

ChatBots: these are used in sports to answer fans' questions on a wide range of topics, including live game information, team statistics, gym and stadium information. They can also help athletes monitor their daily caloric intake, suggest diet plans, and remind them to stay hydrated and take necessary supplements. They can also teach athletes the importance of nutrition in recovery.

Wearable technology: is the general name for technology devices that can be worn by humans and are equipped with smart sensors that track body movements. Examples of wearable technology in the sports world include accelerometers, pedometers and GPS that can be used to measure an athlete's energy expenditure and movement pattern. Wearable technology is usually used to monitor a user's health.

Computer vision: is a field of AI that focuses on enabling computers to interpret and understand the visual world. It involves the development of algorithms and techniques that enable computers to recognize and interpret images and videos.

Automated journalism: is a term used to describe the use of automated software programs to create popular articles otherwise called «automated journalism» or «algorithmic journalism.» In the world of sports, automated journalism is a method that media outlets use to reach their customers interested in sports and increase their revenues through AI-focused automation.

In the next section, we will briefly introduce the concept of biohacking before delving into the trio of biohacking, sports and AI.

BIOHACKING

The goal of do-it-yourself (DIY) biology, also called «biohacking,» is to make biology accessible to non-scientists. Over the past decade, DIY biology has evolved from a small, local initiative to a transnational movement. At its inception in 2008, the movement was in its infancy. According to the main website dedicated to the movement (diybio.org), there are currently more than 100 groups interested in DIY biology around the world, most of which are in Europe and the United States. About half of these groups have their own physical spaces, located in Amsterdam, Lima, Paris or New York, for example. DIY biology has even been featured in documentaries or exhibitions (at the Science Gallery in Dublin, the Medical Museum in Copenhagen, the Science Museum in London, and the Ars Electronica in Linz) and at TEDx conferences (Meyer, Vergnaud, 2020).

Biotechnology was originally used to describe innovative studies or work involving the use of cells, bacteria or other organisms, often in the development of drugs or vaccines. Now, you will find the label 'biotechnology' encompasses technologies designed to interface with human or living tissue, for example implants with embedded technology such as retinal or cochlear implants, as well as wearable devices (e.g., smartwatches or glucose monitors that monitor blood glucose continuously). Biotechnology is a rapidly growing field and is expected to include more and more devices and techniques over time.

At this point we can see a space of integration between AI and biohacking tracking that combines with all the means mentioned above.

LOOKING TO THE FUTURE: DRIVING RESPONSIBLE ADVANCEMENT IN THE TRINITY: SPORTS, IA AND BIOHACKING

More and more athletes are showing that they integrate Biohacking into their personal sphere for the purpose of optimizing their performance, recovery, daily energy levels, nutrition, etc. We can mention a few such as for example Novak Djokovic, Erling Haaland or Iga Swiatek . Such optimization can be applied through the use of various means routinely: through internal devices/materials/substances, wearable or external technology; through hardware or software (e.g., brain-machine interface); or through an intelligent environment (e.g., digital or virtual environments) or in nature (Lindfors, 2023). Considering all the technological elements mentioned above, it will not be entirely surprising to be able to guess the innovative role of AI as the data management pivot and common denominator of such devices.

Looking to the future, professional sports biohacking combined with artificial intelligence promises to radically revolutionize the world of sports. Biohacking, the use of technologies and methodologies to improve human performance, could become even more sophisticated with the integration of AI. Not only because of the shared purpose in terms of performance optimization but also because of their easy integration with wearable technology or other devices consonant with the sports sphere.

Through advanced analysis of biometric and physical performance data, AI could provide athletes with an unprecedented level of personalization in their training and competitive strategies. For example, AI algorithms could process data from wearable devices to provide instant feedback on training, suggesting personalized modifications to optimize performance by making use of modern research.

In addition, AI could be used to develop advanced monitoring systems to prevent injuries by analyzing athletes' movement patterns and identifying potential risks. This could enable athletes to maximize their performance while minimizing the risk of injury.

If we consider the world of respiration or Breathwork in English (Nestor, 2020; McKeown, 2021), it represents an important practice that could revolutionize the way athletes approach their training and competitions. Through the analysis of respiratory data, artificial intelligence could offer athletes a deeper understanding of their breathing patterns and heart rates during physical exertion. This would enable athletes to optimize their breathing, regulate heart rate and maximize oxygen intake, key elements in improving performance and endurance. In addition, AI could provide real-time feedback during training and competition, suggesting modifications in breathing technique to suit the specific needs of the athlete and the situation. Ultimately, the integration of breathwork with artificial intelligence could be an important tool for athletes seeking a competitive edge and optimal performance.

CONCLUSION

In conclusion, the integration of artificial intelligence in sports and biohacking offers a number of benefits and challenges that require balanced attention. Among the positives is the potential to improve athletic performance through advanced biometric data analysis and personalization of training. In addition, the use of AI to prevent injuries can help keep athletes at the peak of their physical capabilities and reduce the risks associated with playing sports. However, there are also downsides to consider, such as concerns about the privacy of athletes' biometric data and the risk of abuse or manipulation of the information collected. In addition, there is a risk that AI may create inequality in access to advanced technologies, favoring more affluent professionals and putting less privileged athletes at a disadvantage. Therefore, it is essential to establish strict regulations and standards to ensure that the use of AI in sports remains fair, rule-compliant, and ethics-centered, balancing potential benefits with privacy protection and fairness in competition.

Alessandro Romagnoli
Psychotherapist and Sport Psychologist
www.oxylab360.com
OxyLab360 Co-Founder
Master Oxygen Advantage
Master Buteyko Clinic
Wim Hof Instructor
Scientific Consultant
PHONE: +39 3393321147
EMAIL: alessandro.romagnoli1990@gmail.com

BIBLIOGRAPHY

Copeland B.J. (2023, Aug. 23). Artificial intelligence. Retrieved 15.07.2023 from https:// www.britannica.com/technology/artificial-intelligence).

Kaya, Fatih. (2023). Artificial Intelligence and Its Use in Sports. - Researchgate

Meyer, M., & Vergnaud, F. (2020). The rise of biohacking: Tracing the emergence and evolution of DIY biology through online discussions. Technological Forecasting and Social Change, 160, 120206.

Carver, L. F. (2024). An Interdisciplinary Approach to Aging, Biohacking and Technology.

Lindfors, A. (2023). Between Self-Tracking and Alternative Medicine: Biomimetic Imaginary in Contemporary Biohacking. *Body & Society*, 1357034X231218413.

Nestor, J., & Nestor, J. (2020). *Breath.* Penguin Random House Audio Publishing Group.

McKeown, P. (2021). *The breathing cure: Develop new habits for a healthier, happier, and longer life.* Humanix Books.

Qi, Y., Sajadi, S. M., Baghaei, S., Rezaei, R., & Li, W. (2024). Digital technologies in sports: Opportunities, challenges, and strategies for safeguarding athlete well-being and competitive integrity in the digital era. *Technology in Society*, 102496.

Desai, V. (2024, April). The Future of Artificial Intelligence in Sports Medicine and Return to Play. In *Seminars in Musculoskeletal Radiology* (Vol. 28, No. 02, pp. 203-212). Thieme Medical Publishers, Inc..

Li, Y. M., Hsieh, C. Y., & Fan, S. N. (2024). A social selection mechanism for sports betting market. *Decision Support Systems, 178*, 114119.

Liu, F., & Hang, X. (2024). Design of artificial intelligence volleyball teaching intelligent assistant system based on artificial muscle integrated optical equipment. *Optical and Quantum Electronics, 56*(3), 455.

Conclusions

Maestro, horrible things happen in the world and I don't know what to do. I get sad. I don't know how to help, I don't want to close my eyes, I feel guilty about being okay when the others suffer..."

The Master replied, «When you go to sleep you turn off all the lights, but you turn on the one in your room. You are in your room, exactly where you need to be at that moment, and there you turn on the light so you are not in the dark. That's the way it is in the world.

If there is war and you are not there, it is simply because you don't have to be there and you are where you are. Turn on your light!

If you have something to share please share.

If you have something valuable to bring to the world, don't delay: do it! If you are wise and can give advice, then what are you waiting for to provide it to the world? If you are beautiful and there are many bad things out there, be even more beautiful.

Be part of the beauty of life.

Beauty, as your poets also claim, will save the world... The Light comes on because there are deserts and seas on earth.

If it was written on your path that you should be part of the water, why does the desert afflict you?

If, on the other hand, it has fallen to you to be deserted, then why do the waters afflict you? Everyone is exactly where he is and where he needs to be.

Call it Karma, Destiny. Purpose-so be it. EVERYTHING IS PERFECT.

In war, not everyone dies. Yet, where there is no war, people die. Those who have to die, die.

Who must live, lives. Why feel guilty?

Or do you decide who lives or who dies? What is your responsibility?

Just do what you have to do.

Remember that's why you came into the world. And that is why you are where you are.

Turn on your light.
Be part of the light, not part of the problem,» Master said.
The world, when it is dark, needs more lights on.
We are the light that illuminates the world through knowledge and awareness, study and deepening.
We are down here to learn, so let's not waste time and keep turning on lights.

Sometimes fate resembles a sandstorm that incessantly changes the direction of the path.
To avoid this, change your gait, as much as the wind will also change in turn to follow you better.
Crossing the seas aboard the Amerigo Vespucci, the Italian Navy's training ship, I learned to sail in all waters and in all weather conditions....
This manual is a logbook: use it wisely.
Always remember that you are the commander of your soul and the captain of your vessel. Your soul, better than any compass, will know which course to take.
Observe it and listen to it.
Be ready if it is necessary to change course and tack the sail again, and immediately the wind will change to match your pace.
What seemed like a headwind to you, impossible to rise even with a narrow upwind, will turn into a tailwind.
This is repeated countless times, like a sinister dance with the God of Death before dawn. Because that wind is not something that came from afar, independent of you, but something inside you. That wind is you.
So the only thing you can do is to get into it, into that wind. Sail into the wind, let the sails swell up and close your eyes tightly, if need be, so as not to let sea water into the hold...

Bibliography

Olusanya B.O., Kaplan M., Hansen T.W.R. Neonatal hyperbilirubinemia: A global perspective. Lancet Child Adolesc. Health. 2018; 2:610-620. doi: 10.1016/S2352-4642(18)30139-1. - DOI - PubMed

Anupriya K.S., Pradeep N. Cord blood albumin level as a predictor of neonatal physiological jaundice in healthy term neonate. Indian J. Child Health. 2023; 10:77-79. doi: 10.32677/ijch.v10i6.3998. - DOI

Gao C., Guo Y., Huang M., He J., Qiu X. Breast Milk Constituents and the Development of Breast Milk Jaundice in Neonates: A Systematic Review. Nutrients. 2023; 15:2261. doi: 10.3390/nu15102261. - DOI - PMC - PubMed

Kumar V., Kumar P., Sundaram V., Munjal S.K., Malhi P., Panda N.K. Childhood neurodevelopmental outcomes of survivors of acute bilirubin encephalopathy: A retrospective cohort study. Early Hum. Dev. 2021;158:105380. doi: 10.1016/j.earlhumdev.2021.105380. - DOI - PubMed

Wang J., Guo G., Li A., Cai W.Q., Wang X. Challenges of phototherapy for neonatal hyperbilirubinemia (Review) Exp. Ther. Med. 2021; 21:231. DOI: 10.3892/etm.2021.9662. - DOI - PMC - PubMed

ADSC and tissue regeneration N. Naderi et al. Acknowledgements We would like to thank Belinda Colton MSc for coloring of ADSCs in Figure 1, Douglas Neil for designing Figure 2 and Steve Atherton MA RMIP MIMI for designing Figure 3.

Mizuno H. Adipose-derived stem cells for tissue repair and regeneration: ten years of research and a literature review. J Nippon Med 2009; 76 :56-66.

Zuk PA, Zhu M, Mizuno H, Huang J, Futrell JW, Katz AJ, Benhaim PH, Lorenz P, Hedrick MH. Multilineage cells from human adipose tissue: implications for cell-based therapies. Tissue Eng 2001;

Zuk PA. The adipose-derived stem cell: looking back and looking ahead. Mol Biol Cell 2010;21:1783-7.

Watson D, Keller GS, Lacombe V, Fodor PB, Rawnsley J, Lask GP. Autologous fibroblasts for treatment of facial rhytids and dermal depressions. A pilot study. Arch

Facial Plast Surg 1999;
11 Lenoir N. Europe confronts the embryonic stem cell research challenge. Science 2000;287:1425-7.

Ben-David U, Benvenisty N. The tumorigenicity of human embryonic and induced pluripotent stem cells. Nat Rev Cancer 2011; 11:268-77.

Dodson MV, Hausman GJ, Guan L, Du M, Rasmussen TP, Poulos SP, Mir P, Bergen WG, Fernyhough ME, McFarland DC, Rhoads RP, Soret B, Reecy JM, Velleman SG, Jiang Z. Skeletal muscle stem cells from animals I. Basic cell biology. Int J Biol Sci 2010;6:465-74.

Belicchi M, Pisati F, Lopa R, Porretti L, Fortunato F, Sironi M, Scalamonga M, Parati EA, Bresolin N, Torrente Y. Human skin-derived stem cells migrate throughout forebrain and differentiate into astrocytes after injection into adult mouse brain. J. Neurosci Res 2004;77:475-86.

Feng J, Mantesso A, Sharpe PT. Perivascular cells as mesenchymal stem cells. Expert Opin Biol Ther 2010;10:1441

Shi M, Ishikawa M, Kamei N, Nakasa T, Adachi N, Deie M, Asahara T, Ochi M. Acceleration of skeletal muscle regeneration in a rat skeletal muscle injury model by local injection of human peripheral blood-derived CD133-positive cells. Stem Cells 2009;27:949-60.

Miura M, Gronthos S, Zhao M, Lu B, Fisher LW, Robey PG, Shi S. SHED: stem cells from human exfoliated deciduous teeth. Proc Natl Acad Sci U S A 2003;100:5807-12.

Seo B-M, Miura M, Gronthos S, Bartold PM, Batouli S, Brahim J, Young M, Robey PG, Wang CY, Shi S. Investigation of multipotent postnatal stem cells from human periodontal ligament. Lancet 2004;364:149-55.

Baksh D, Yao R, Tuan RS. Comparison of proliferative and multilineage differentiation potential of human mesenchymal stem cells derived from umbilical cord and bone marrow. Stem Cells 2007;25:1384-92.

Musina RA, Bekchanova ES, Sukhikh GT. Comparison of mesenchymal stem cells obtained from different human tissues. Bull Exp Biol Med 2005; 139 :504-9.

Zuk PA, Zhu M, Ashjian P, De Ugarte DA, Huang JI, Mizuno H, Alfonso ZC, Fraser JK,

Benhaim P, Hedrick MH. Human adipose tissue is a source of multipotent stem cells. Mol Biol Cell 2002;13:4279-95.

Gimble JM, Katz AJ, Bunnell BA. Adipose-derived stem cells for regenerative medicine. Circ Res 2007;100:1249-60.

Tobita M, Orbay H, Mizuno H. Adipose-derived stem cells: current findings and future perspectives. Discov Med 2011;11:160-70.

Yoshimura K, Sato K, Aoi N, Kurita M, Hirohi T, Harii K. Cell-assisted lipotransfer for cosmetic breast augmentation: supportive use of adipose derived stem/stromal cells. Aesthetic Plast Surg 2008; 32:48-55; disc. 56-7.

Khalifian S, Sarhane KA, Tammia M, Ibrahim Z, Mao H-Q, Cooney DS, Shores JT, Lee WPA, Brandacher G. Stem cell-based approaches to improve nerve regeneration: potential implications for reconstructive transplantation? Arch Immunol Ther Exp (Warsz) 2015;63:15-30.

Marino G, Moraci M, Armenia E, Orabona C, Sergio R, De Sena G, Capuozzo V, Barbarisi M, Rosso F, Giordano G, Iovino F, Bargarisi A. Therapy with autologous adipose-derived regenerative cells for the care of chronic ulcer of lower limbs in patients with peripheral arterial disease. J Surg Res 2013; 185:36-44.

Gronthos S, Franklin DM, Leddy HA, Robey PG, Storms RW, Gimble JM. Surface protein characterization of human adipose tissue-derived stromal cells. J Cell Physiol 2001;189:54-63.

De Ugarte DA, Morizono K, Elbarbary A, Alfonso Z, Zuk PA, Zhu M, Dragoo JL, Ashjian P, Thomas B, Benhaim P, Chen I, Fraser J, Hedrick MH. Comparison of multi-lineage cells from human adipose tissue and bone marrow. Cells Tissues Organs 2003;174:101-9.

Wagner W, Wein F, Seckinger A, Frankhauser M, Wirkner U, Krause U, Blake J, Schwager C, Eckstein V, Ansorge W, Ho AD. Comparative characteristics of mesenchymal stem cells from human bone marrow, adipose tissue, and umbilical cord blood. Exp Hematol 2005;33:1402-16.

Kern S, Eichler H, Stoeve J, Klüter H, Bieback K. Comparative analysis of mesenchymal stem cells from bone marrow, umbilical cord blood, or adipose tissue. Stem Cells 2006;24:1294-301.

Fraser JK, Wulur I, Alfonso Z, Hedrick MH. Fat tissue: an underappreciated source of stem cells for biotechnology. Trends Biotechnol 2006;24:150-4.

McIntosh K, Zvonic S, Garrett S, Mitchell JB, Floyd ZE, Hammill L, Kloster A, Di Halvorsen Y, Ting JP, Storms RW, Goh B, Kilroy G, Wu X, Gimble JM. The immunogenicity of human adipose-derived cells: temporal changes in vitro. Stem Cells 2006;24:1246-53.

Mitchell JB, McIntosh K, Zvonic S, Garrett S, Floyd ZE, Kloster A, Di Halvorsen Y, Storms RW, Goh RW, Kilroy G, Wu X, Gimble JM. Immunophenotype of human adipose-derived cells: temporal changes in stromal-associated and stem cell-associated markers. Stem Cells 2006;24:376-85.

Zimmerlin L, Donnenberg VS, Pfeifer ME, Meyer EM, Péault B, Rubin JP, Donnenberg AD. Stromal vascular progenitors in adult human adipose tissue. Cytometry A 2010;77:22-30.

Pachón-Peña G, Yu G, Tucker A, Wu X, Vendrell J, Bunnell BA, Gimble JM. Stromal stem cells from adipose tissue and bone marrow of age-matched female donors display distinct immunophenotypic profiles. J Cell Physiol 2011;226:843-51.

Planat-Benard V, Silvestre J-S, Cousin B, André M, Nibbelink M, Tamarat R, Clergue M, Manneville C, Saillan-Barreau C, Duriez M, Tedgui A, Levy B, Penicaud L, Casteilla L. Plasticity of human adipose lineage cells toward endothelial cells: physiological and therapeutic perspectives. Circulation 2004;109:656-63.

Konno M, Hamazaki TS, Fukuda S, Tokuhara M, Uchiyama H, Okazawa H, Okochi H, Asashima M. Efficiently differentiating vascular endothelial cells from adipose tissue-derived mesenchymal stem cells in serum-free culture. Biochem Biophys Res Commun 2010;400:461-5.

Rangappa S, Fen C, Lee EH, Bongso A, Sim EKW, Wei EKS. Transformation of adult mesenchymal stem cells isolated from the fatty tissue into cardiomyocytes. Ann Thorac Surg 2003;75:775.

The Cyborg Foundation https://www.cyborgfoundation.com/
«The Cyborg Foundation is an online platform for the research, development and promotion of project Related To The Creation Of New Senses And Perceptions By Applying Technology To The Human Body. Our Mission Is To Help People Become Cyborgs, Promote Cyborg Art And Defend Cyborg Rights.»

New York Times article on «A Do-it-yourself revolution in Diabetes Care «Retrieved June 12, 2019. https://www.nytimes.com/2016/02/23/health/a-do-it-yourself- revolution-in-diabetes-care.html

Retrieved June 12, 2019 https://hackernoon.com/biohack-your- intelligence-now-or-become-obsolete-97cdd15e395f

https://hackernoon.com/im-32-and-spent-200k-on-biohacking- became-calmer-thinner-extroverted-healthier-happier-2a2e846ae113

Retrieved June 12 2019 June 5 2018 by Faye Flam «it is not illegal to experiment on yourself FDA»

https://www.bloomberg.com/opinion/articles/2018-06-05/ biohackers-experimenting-on-themselves-new-drugs-old-technique Bloomberg: Warning: Don't Try This Biohacking At Home. Early this year, a 28-year-old self-described biohacker named Aaron Traywick injected himself with an alleged herpes vaccine prepared by fellow amateur medical researchers. The injection, which was broadcast on Facebook Live, brought on a volley of criticism and ethical concerns. Only a few months earlier, a colleague at the company Traywick founded, Ascendance Biomedical, injected himself with an alleged gene therapy for HIV. It's unlikely either of these treatments worked, but they succeeded in proving how easy it's become for amateurs to experiment with infectious agents and other biological materials that were once restricted to trained professionals. While it's illegal to sell biohacked therapies or vaccines, or to test them on human subjects, so far at least, the FDA does not explicitly forbid experimenting on yourself.

Brain interfaces for paralyzed patients since 2006 https://www.nytimes.com/2006/07/13/science/13brain.html

New England Journal of Medicine
Fully Implanted Brain-Computer Interface in a Locked-In Patient with ALS https://www.nejm.org/doi/full/10.1056/NEJMoa1608085 July 7 2013
Retrieved on June 14, 2019

https://io9.gizmodo.com/what-you-need-to-know-about-getting- magnetic-finger-imp-813537993

Hacklab Toronto Retrieved June 13, 2019 https://hacklab.to/

Eric Boyd Cyborg - Canadian https://ca.linkedin.com/in/eric-boyd-2b5ab83

http://makerfestival.ca/team/eric-boyd/
Eric Boyd is the founder of Sensebridge, an electronic jewelry company. Born and raised in Ontario Canada on a small chicken farm, Eric went to Queens University for engineering, graduating in 2003, but not before co-founding StumbleUpon.com. After graduating, he lived and worked in Silicon Valley at a high tech startup, designing and installing industrial sensors. Eric is currently based in Toronto Canada, where he is President of Hacklab.to, a technology community space and a trustee of the Awesome Foundation. At Sensebridge, Eric works on a variety of devices which are intended to augment the user, turning them into a cyborg. These devices include North Paw, a compass anklet that gives users a sense of direction, and Heart Spark, a heart-beat flashing pendant which broadcasts the wearers emotions. A man of diverse interests, his other hobbies include Quantified Self, DIYbio and Guerrilla Gardening.
Neil Harbisson had an antenna implanted into his skull so he could see colors.

Commentary on: Photobiomodulation: The Clinical Applications of Low Level Light Therapy. Sun Y, et al. Aesthet Surg J. 2021. PMID: 33647952 No abstract available.

Photobiomodulation: A review of the molecular evidence for low level light therapy. Glass GE. J Plast Reconstr Aesthet Surg. 2021. PMID: 33436333 Review.

Low-level laser (light) therapy (LLLT) in skin: stimulating, healing, restoring. Avci P, et al. Semin Cutan Med Surg. 2013. PMID: 24049929 Free PMC article. Review.

Photobiomodulation with 808-nm diode laser light promotes wound healing of human endothelial cells through increased reactive oxygen species production stimulating mitochondrial oxidative phosphorylation. Amaroli A, et al. Lasers Med Sci. 2019. PMID: 30145725

Photobiomodulation: A Systematic Review of the Oncologic Safety of Low-Level Light Therapy for Aesthetic Skin Rejuvenation. Glass GE. Aesthet Surg J. 2023. PMID: 36722207 Free PMC article.

Low-level laser therapy for wound healing: mechanism and efficacy. Posten W, et al. Dermatol Surg. 2005. PMID: 15841638 Review.

Reverse skin aging signs by red light photobiomodulation. Couturaud V, et al. Skin Res Technol. 2023. PMID: 37522497 Free PMC article.

The effect of different treatment protocols with diode laser on regeneration in axonetmesis ınjuries of the ınferior alveolar nerve: an animal study. Öztürk K, et al. Lasers Med Sci. 2023. PMID: 37515606

The Effects and Mechanisms of PBM Therapy in Accelerating Orthodontic Tooth Movement. Wang X, et al. Biomolecules. 2023. PMID: 37509176 Free PMC article. Review.

Male facial rejuvenation using a combination 633, 830, and 1072 nm LED face mask. Mineroff J., et al. Arch Dermatol Res. 2023. PMID: 37418018

Effect of photobiomodulation in addition to periodontal therapy on individuals with type 2 diabetes mellitus regarding periodontal clinical parameters: a systematic review and meta-analysis. Freire BL, et al. Laser Med Sci. 2023. PMID: 37140820

In Shape in Three Weeks. Unleash your innate potential. Adolfo
Panfili, Valeria Mangani, Tecniche Nuove Editions, June 2012

Nutrigenomics, Blood Groups and Diet. Adolfo Panfili, Valeria Mangani, Tecniche Nuove Editions, March 2011

Blood Groups and Diet. How to guard against food intolerances and develop the therapeutic power of your blood group. Adolfo Panfili, Valeria Mangani, Tecniche Nuove Editions, August 2005

The Diet for the Soul. Adolfo Panfili, Valeria Mangani, Tecniche Nuove Editions, January 2004

Candida, the silent epidemic: allergy of the 20th century? Preventing and treating it with Orthomolecular Medicine. Adolfo Panfili, Valeria Mangani, Tecniche Nuove Editions, January 2000

pH and the Orthomolecular Diet. Basic acid balance, a foundation of health. Adolfo Panfili, Valeria Mangani, Tecniche Nuove Editions, January 2000

Orthomolecular medicine. A therapy on a human scale. Adolfo Panfili, Valeria Mangani, Tecniche Nuove Editions, January 2000

The pH diet. Measure your pH for orthomolecular health of body, mind and soul. Adolfo Panfili, Valeria Mangani, Tecniche Nuove Editions, April 2006

The Poison Tooth. «The Toxic Metal Syndrome and the Toxicity Riddle of Dental Amalgams.» Adolfo Panfili, Tecniche Nuove Editions, January 2000

Khavinson et al. Peptide Bioregulation of aging, results and prospects Biogerontology volume11, pages139-149(2010)

Amanda Rosenthal, Ronald Moy. The role of bioidentical hormone replacement therapy in anti-aging Medicine: a review of the literature (2020)

Peter L.J. de Keizer. The Fountain of Youth by Targeting Senescent Cells?

Rafik Salama, Mahito Sadaie, Matthew Hoare, and Masashi Narita - Cellular senescence and its effector programs GENES & DEVELOPMENT 28:99-114 Published by Cold Spring Harbor Laboratory Press

Laura Forcina, Carmen Miano, Bianca Maria Scicchitano, Antonio Musarò Review Signals from the Niche: Insights into the Role of IGF-1 and IL-6 in Modulating Skeletal Muscle Fibrosis (2019)

Junilla RK, List EO, Berryman DE,et al. The GH/IGF-1 axis in aging and longevity. Nat Rev Endocrinol. 2013

Minireview: Mechano-Growth Factor: A Putative Product of IGF-I Gene Expression Involved in Tissue Repair and Regeneration Ronald W. Matheny Endocrinology 151: 865-875, 2010

Goldspink G, et al. Gene expression in skeletal muscle in response to mechanical signs. Am J Physiol1992; 262: R326-63

Laura Forcina, Carmen Miano, Bianca Maria Scicchitano, Antonio Musarò Review Signals from the Niche: Insights into the Role of IGF-1 and IL-6 in Modulating Skeletal Muscle Fibrosis (2019)

Lalancette-Hebert M, Gowing G, Simard A, Weng YC, Kriz J. Selective ablation of proliferating microglia cells exacerbates ischemic injury in the brain. J Neurosci 2007;27: 2596-2605

Jeon, S. G., Hong, S. B., Nam, Y., Tae, J., Yoo, A., Ji Song, E., Moon, M. (2019).
Ghrelin in Alzheimer's disease: pathologic roles and therapeutic implications. Ageing Research Reviews

Johannes D. Veldhuis (2009) Determinants of GH-releasing hormone and GH-releasing peptide synergy in men Am J Physiol Endocrinol Metab 296: E1085-E1092

Tomas, A. Lemmey Superior potency of infused IGF-I analogues which bind poorly to IGF-binding proteins is maintained when administered by injection. DOI:10.1677/joe.0.1500077 (1996)

Mac E Hadley 1, Discovery that a melanocortin regulates sexual functions in male and female humans -Peptides - 2005 Oct;26(10):1687-9. doi: 10.1016/j

H Wessells. Melanocortin receptor agonists, penile erection, and sexual motivation: human studies with Melanotan II - International Journal of Impotence Research (2000)

Li, Juan Jenny et al. «Thymosin alpha 1: Biological activities, applications and genetic engineering production.» Peptides 31 (2010): 2151-2158.

Essential Bibliography of Adolfo Panfili

Adolfo Panfili, Valeria Mangani
Get in Shape in Three Weeks
Unleash Your Innate Potential
Tecniche Nuove, June 2012

Adolfo Panfili, Valeria Mangani
Nutrigenomics, Blood Groups, and Diet
Tecniche Nuove, January 2011

Adolfo Panfili, Valeria Mangani
The pH Diet
Measure Your pH for the Orthomolecular Health of the Body, Mind, and Soul
Tecniche Nuove, April 2006

Adolfo Panfili, Valeria Mangani
Blood Groups and Diet
How to Defend Yourself from Food Intolerances and Develop the Therapeutic Power of Your Blood Type
Tecniche Nuove, August 2005

Adolfo Panfili, Valeria Mangani
The Diet for the Soul
Tecniche Nuove, January 2004

Adolfo Panfili, Valeria Mangani
pH and Orthomolecular Diet
Acid-Base Balance, a Foundation of Health
Tecniche Nuove, September 2000

Adolfo Panfili
Orthomolecular Medicine
A Human-Centered Therapy
Tecniche Nuove, August 1995

Adolfo Panfili, Valeria Mangani
Candida, the Silent Epidemic: Allergy of the 20th Century?
How to Prevent and Treat It with Orthomolecular Medicine
Tecniche Nuove, September 1996

Adolfo Panfili
The Poisoned Tooth
Toxic Metal Syndrome and the Riddle of Dental Amalgam Toxicity
Tecniche Nuove, October 2000

QR Codes

Dreamers Day 2017

Prof. Adolfo Panfili

Prof. Adolfo Panfili in conversation with Francesca Del Nero

"Orthomolecular Nutrition: conscious feeding" Interview with Adolfo Panfili at Rete55

Prof. Adolfo Panfili: Cervical disc hernia

Disc herniation with minimally invasive technique - OneMorning 2010 - Prof. Adolfo Panfili

Turn your vocation into a vacation to be successful for weight loss

Let's talk about stem cells with Professor Adolfo Panfili

Archetypes of life with Prof. Adolfo Panfili

End of Academic Year

The science of Orthomolecular medicine, it's a Rubik's cube.

Powerful Meditation For The Mind. Guided Meditation By Gurudev Sri Sri Ravi Shankar

Orthomolecular Biohacking is the alchemical fusion of Prof. Panfili between science and nature, where the molecules of the Earth merge with human technologies to create a new level of health and well-being.

It is a synthesis of ancestral knowledge and modern innovations, where nature intertwines with AI.

It is a futuristic vision in which man and nature come together to transcend limits and achieve a level of health and human potential never reached before.

FOR INFO ON TRAINING ACTIVITIES, VISITS, WEB CONSULTATIONS CONTACT:
HYPERLINK "mailto:aimo@aimo.it"aimo@aimo.it - +393339605191

Finito di stampare nel mese di luglio 2024

Made in the USA
Monee, IL
05 November 2026

67810732R00174